Case Studies in Stroke

Neurologists learn from their patients, and this selection of 60 stroke cases will inform and challenge clinicians at all stages in their careers. Including both common and unusual cases, the aim is to reinforce diagnostic skills through careful analysis of individual presenting patterns, and to guide treatment decisions. Each case consists of a clinical history, examination findings and special investigations, usually involving imaging before a diagnosis is given. There then follows for each case a discussion of the clinical issues raised by the case, in which the main teaching points are emphasized. Selected references, frequently including the first description, are provided at the conclusion of each case.

Drawing on the expertise of leading teachers and practitioners, and liberally illustrated, these case studies and the discussions that accompany them are an essential guide to learning the complexity of stroke diagnosis.

Michael G. Hennerici is Professor of Neurology at the University of Heidelberg, and Chairman at the Department of Neurology, University Hospital in Mannheim, and the editor, with Stephen Meairs, of *Cerebrovascular Ultrasound; Theory, Practice and Future Developments*, published by Cambridge University Press. He is Chairman of the European Stroke Conference.

Michael Daffertshofer is Professor of Neurology at the University of Heidelberg, and former Director of the Stroke Unit, University Hospital in Mannheim.

Louis Caplan is Professor of Neurology at Harvard Medical School and Senior Neurologist at Beth Israel Deaconess Medical Center, Boston. He is the editor, with Julien Bogousslavsky, of *Stroke Syndromes* and *Uncommon Causes of Stroke*, both published by Cambridge University Press.

Kristina Szabo is Senior Lecturer at the University of Heidelberg, University Hospital in Mannheim and the MR-Neurology Research Unit, and is an expert in neuroimaging.

Case Studies in Stroke

Common and Uncommon Presentations

Michael G. Hennerici, M.D.

Department of Neurology
Universitätsklinikum Mannheim
University of Heidelberg
Germany

Michael Daffertshofer, M.D.

Department of Neurology
Universitätsklinikum Mannheim
University of Heidelberg
Germany

Louis R. Caplan, M.D.

Cerebrovascular Division
Beth Israel Deaconess Medical Center
Harvard Medical School, USA

Kristina Szabo, M.D.

Department of Neurology
Universitätsklinikum Mannheim
University of Heidelberg
Germany

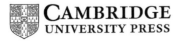

CAMBRIDGE
UNIVERSITY PRESS

CAMBRIDGE UNIVERSITY PRESS
Cambridge, New York, Melbourne, Madrid, Cape Town, Singapore, São Paulo

Cambridge University Press
The Edinburgh Building, Cambridge CB2 2RU, UK

Published in the United States of America by Cambridge University Press, New York

www.cambridge.org
Information on this title: www.cambridge.org/9780521673679

First published 2007

Printed in the United Kingdom at the University Press, Cambridge

A catalog record for this publication is available from the British Library

ISBN-13 978-0-521-67367-9 paperback
ISBN-10 0-521-67367-4 paperback

To our friends and colleagues in the Department of Neurology, University Hospital, Mannheim, Ruprecht-Karls-University of Heidelberg, who contributed to this book. We gratefully acknowledge their daily enthusiasm and dedication to treat stroke patients, who teach us how to better meet their needs.

Contents

The following cases described herein have been published previously

Case 8   Lanczik, O., Szabo, K., Gass, A., & Hennerici, M. G. Tinnitus after cycling. *Lancet* 2003; **362**:292.

Case 13   Amoiridis, G., Wöhrle, J. C., Langkafel, M., Maiwurm, D., & Przuntek, H. Spinal cord infarction after surgery in a patient in the hyperlordotic position. *Anesthesiology* 1996; **84**:228–230.

Case 14   Lie, C., Schwenk, S., Szabo, K., Lanczik, O., Hennerici, M. G., & Gass, A. Bilateral internal carotid artery dissection mimicking inflammatory demyelinating disease. *J. Neuroimaging* 2003; **13**:359–361.

Case 17   Sedlaczek, O., Grips, E., Bäzner, H., Claus, A., Wöhrle, J., & Hennerici, M. Infarction of the central cerebellar arbor vitae and transient loss of spatial orientation. *Neurology* 2005; **65**:168.

Case 18   Binder, J., Pfleger, S., & Schwarz, S. Images in cardiovascular medicine. Right atrial primary cardiac lymphoma presenting with stroke. *Circulation* 2004; **110**:e451–452.

Case 25   Szabo, K., Gass, A., Rossmanith, C., Hirsch, J. G., & Hennerici, M. G. Diffusion- and perfusion-weighted MRI demonstrates synergistic lesions in acute ischemic Foix–Chavany–Marie syndrome. *J. Neurol.* 2002; **249**:1735–1737.

Case 32   Sommer, A., Meairs, S., Gueckel, F., Cornelius, A., & Schwartz, A. Traumatic brachiocephalic pseudoaneurysm presenting with delayed stroke: case report. *Neuroradiology* 2000; **42**:742–745.

Case 36   Kern, R., Kreisel, S., Zoubaa, S., Szabo, K., Gass, A., & Hennerici, M. Cognitive impairment, aphasia, and seizures in a 51-year-old man. *Lancet Neurol.* 2005; **4**:445–450.

Case 52   Gass, A. & Hennerici, M. G. MRI of basilar-artery-aneurysm growth. *Lancet Neurol.* 2003; **2**:128.

Contributors

Hansjörg Bäzner, M.D.

Rolf Kern, M.D.

Johannes Binder, M.D.

Achim Gass, M.D.

Oliver Sedlaczek, M.D.

Stefan Schwarz, M.D.

Christian Blahak, M.D.

Martin Griebe, M.D.

Christian Sick, M.D.

Johannes Wöhrle, M.D.

Tobias Back, M.D.

Simone Bukow, M.D.

Anastasios Chatzikonstantinou, M.D.

Yaroslav Epifanov, M.D.

Marc Fatar, M.D.

Alex Förster, M.D.

Bianca Götz, M.D.

Eva Grips, M.D.

Micha Kablau, M.D.

Anne-Christine Karow, M.D.

Stefan Kreisel, M.D.

Oliver Lanczik, M.D.

Stephen Meairs, M.D.

Christian Peters, M.D.

Yogesh Shah, M.D.

Abbreviations

ACA	anterior cerebral artery
ADC	apparent diffusion coefficient (MRI)
aCH	acetylcholine
ADEM	acute disseminated encephalomyelitis
AO	aorta
APL	antiphospholipid antibodies
aPTT	activated partial thromboplastin time
ASD	atrial septal defect
AVM	arteriovenous malformation
CAA	cerebral amyloid angioplasty
CBF	cerebral blood flow
CBS	cystathionine beta synthetase
CCF	carotid cavernous fistula
CRP	C-reactive protein
CSF	cerebrospinal fluid
CCT	cranial computed tomography
CT	computed tomography
CTA	computed tomography angiography
CVT	cerebral venous thrombosis
CWS	capsular warning syndrome (Donnan syndrome)
DCS	decompression sickness
DVT	deep vein thrombosis
DWI	diffusion-weighted imaging (MRI)
ECASS	European Cooperative Acute Stroke Study
ECD	extracranial Doppler
ECG	electrocardiogram
EEG	electroencephalography
EP	evoked potential
FCMS	Foix–Chavany–Marie syndrome
FLAIR	fluid attenuated inversion recovery (MRI)
fMRI	functional MRI
GCS	Glasgow Coma Score

HITS	high intensity transient signals (Doppler sonography)
ICA	internal carotid artery
ICH	intracerebral hemorrhage
ICU	intensive care unit
INR	international normalized ratio
MCA	middle cerebral artery
MRA	magnetic resonance angiography
MRI	magnetic resonance imaging
NIHSS	National Institute of Health Stroke Scale
NVAF	non-valvular atrial fibrillation
PCA	posterior cerebral artery
PE	pulmonary embolism
PET	positron emission tomography
PFO	patent foramen ovale
PICA	posterior inferior cerebellar artery
PWI	perfusion-weighted imaging (MRI)
RCTs	randomized clinical trials
rt-PA	recombinant tissue plasminogen activator
SAH	subarachnoid hemorrhage
SVE	subcortical vascular encephalopathy
TCD	transcranial Doppler sonography
TEE	transesophageal echocardiography
TGA	transient global amnesia
TIA	transient ischemic attack
VA	vertebral artery
WML	white matter lesions

Preface

Despite increasing research interest in basic neurosciences, and through random-ised clinical trials, case reports remain the daily experience of academic phys-icians. Stroke is an important and rapidly growing field in neurology and beyond, placing a large burden on patients, relatives and the economy in industrialized societies. Widely disregarded a quarter of a century ago, the diagnostics of brain tissue and vascular structures and classification of stroke subtypes, pro-gnosis and outcome have improved considerably. This has led to better manage-ment through very early, specific treatment on stroke units, as well as primary and secondary prevention strategies in subjects at risk. Interdisciplinary work amongst neurologists, who generally lead the stroke team, cardiologists, neuro-surgeons, interventional radiologists and physiotherapists, speech therapists, rehabilitation and preventive medicine physicians has created a widespread stroke network around the world. Supported by academic grants, a large scientific community is now involved in international research, and major stroke confer-ences attract thousands of attendees to exchange their ideas, from bench-to-bedside and vice versa.

Despite these worldwide, interdisciplinary activities, physicians, and neurolo-gists in particular, still enjoy the challenge of evaluating patients who present with diagnostic and therapeutic difficulties. This is reflected by the continued popularity of *Case Histories* and *Case Reports* during the *European Stroke Confer-ence* as well as their presentation in major leading world journals. This is line with earlier authors in stroke history, from the seventeenth century (e.g. J.J. Wepfer and T. Willis) to the present day (e.g. C. Miller-Fisher and J. Marshall), who have contributed to our current understanding based on meticulous history taking and tireless commitment to their patients. Following in their footsteps, members of the Department of Neurology, Mannheim, collected 60 cases, some of which have already been published previously, offering a range of informative presenta-tions with an emphasis of critical aspects in history, examination, investigations, therapeutic decisions, secondary prevention or rehabilitation. Just enough infor-mation has been presented in the title of each case (see Contents) to attract the reader's attention without providing give-away clues or a definite diagnosis or management advice if possible. Once the reader has made up his own mind, he may turn the page and read a brief commentary or summary of the case, accompanied by a short list of references including early descriptions and recent reviews or controversies of the condition discussed as far as they are available. For an outside opinion, Louis Caplan from Harvard Medical School, one of the pioneers of clinical stroke research, kindly agreed to read all the cases carefully, discuss specific aspects in detail as he has been used to throughout his career and suggest occasional re-writing.

These cases are aimed at improving the knowledge of all our medical colleagues interested in stroke. Students and residents will find the exercises in topical and functional diagnosis in common cases of stroke stimulating. The cases are designed to check their individual expertise and knowledge. Physicians with greater neurological expertise will hopefully appreciate the presentation of un-common cases and may recall similar cases that have challenged them in the past. This book will have achieved its goal if readers at any stage of their career enjoy reading, discussing and following up some of our ideas and thoughts to the benefit of treating their own patients.

Stroke neurology probably represents a unique medical speciality, where sys-tematic thinking based on highly sophisticated neuroanatomy and neurophysi-ology, and expressed through clinical examination and investigative findings, finds its way into more general medical disciplines. Neurologists are traditionally experts in addressing pathophysiology and differential diagnosis, and are still fascinated by extremely rare illnesses despite serving regularly in emergency and intensive care teams.

We follow the specific techniques of neurology in crystallizing all elements of a complex case into a few informative sentences to help students and residents to increase their skills of analytic listening to the history and the clinical findings. We attempt to quickly localize the site of the lesion, deduce the probable pathophysiological process, formulate a differential diagnosis and estimate the prognosis and outcome once treatment decisions have been established. This approach has been used for all the cases of this book, as it reflects daily practice and is considered to be effective in other disciplines as well.

We gratefully acknowledge the cooperation of the internal medicine physicians, neuroradiologists, neurosurgeons, psychologists and radiologists as well as our emergency and intensive care colleagues in the Universitätsklinikum Mannheim, University of Heidelberg for their continuous support in the care of stroke patients. Some of the cases presented clearly carry their signature, enthusiasm and input in providing and interpreting data and figures collected. Furthermore, we appreciate the careful and continuous support of our secretaries, Birgit Fleig, Maria Garcia-Knapp, and Erika Schneider, in preparing the manuscript and necessary preparation of the book. We offer special thanks to the staff of

Cambridge University Press for their general support and their meticulous editorial work. Last but not least, we are most grateful to our families and partners – without their love and support this book would not have been possible.

We hope that readers will enjoy these cases and that the lessons learned will assist them in providing better care for their patients.

Michael Hennerici
Michael Daffertshofer
Louis Caplan
Kristina Szabo

Introduction: Approach to the patient

It happened on April 13, 1737, as "the whole house vibrated from a dull thud . . . something huge and heavy must have crashed down on the upper floor." The servant of the composer George Frederick Handel ran up the stairs to his master's workroom and found him "lying lifeless on the floor, eyes staring open . . ." Handel had come home from the rehearsal in a furious rage, his face bright red, his temples pulsating. He had slammed the house door and then stamped about, as the servant could hear, on the first floor back and forth so that the ceiling rebounded: it wasn't advisable, on such anger-filled days, to be casual in your service.

From the lower floor Christopher Smith, the master's assistant, went upstairs; he had also been shocked by the thud. He ran to fetch the doctor for the royal composer. "How old is he?" "Fifty-two," answered Smith. "Terrible age, he had worked like an ox." Dr. Jenkins bent deeply over him. "He is, however, strong as an ox. Now we will see what he can do." He noticed that one eye, the right one, stared lifeless and the other one reacted. He tried to lift the right arm. It fell back lifeless. He then lifted the left one. The left one stayed in the new position. Now Dr. Jenkins knew enough. As he left the room, Smith followed him to the stairs, worried. "What is it?" "Apoplexia. The right side is paralysed." "And will . . ."- Smith formed the words – "will he recover?" Dr. Jenkins laboriously took a pinch of snuff. He didn't like such questions. "Perhaps. Anything is possible."

This colorful excerpt from the famous story *George Frederick Handel's Resurrection* by Stefan Zweig illustrates a long-lasting dilemma for doctor and patient after an acute stroke: the question of diagnosis and prognosis.

Today, 260 years after George Frederick Handel's stroke, Dr. Jenkins' successors are better informed about the pathomechanisms involved in the acute situation, for example, ischemia vs. hemorrhage, cardio- and arterioembolic vs. hemodynamic sources of ischemia, or small-vessel vs. large-vessel disease. Even less common etiologies can be identified by additional tests (e.g., cerebrospinal fluid, biologic and immunologic tests). The benefits of acute therapy with a view to the different aetiologies have risen, and the prognosis can be more accurately estimated: Small cerebral hemorrhages or lacunar ischemic lesions have a good prognosis, both being related to chronic, often inadequately treated, hypertension in patients with subcortical vascular encephalopathy; this was most likely the cause of Handel's stroke. We also have begun to elucidate the mechanisms of recovery after stroke. Functional magnetic resonance and studies with positron emission tomography have shown that, following ischemic damage to either cerebral hemisphere, residual connections to corresponding remote areas can be activated and that even new synapses and neural network transformations are possible. These new findings have updated previous misconceptions regarding lack of plasticity in the adult human brain. Many of these new techniques have limited the application of our nearly outdated traditional tests (e.g., conventional angiography).

Nevertheless, the clinical case still presents a challenge for our colleagues in medicine, whether they are students, residents or physicians with advanced expertise in stroke care. Like Dr. Jenkins generations of physicians and neurologists in particular have based their diagnosis on a combination of (a) *temporal profiles* of illnesses, and (b) the presence or absence of focal, symmetric, common, or uncommon *signs and symptoms* of stroke to conclude on the likely pathogenesis and pathobiology. The editors and contributors of this book have tried to crystallize a series of common and uncommon stroke cases and to discuss key elements, whether they are clinical, brain and vascular imaging derived or of other types of individual work-up. Beyond traditional concepts and performance, the actual principle "time is brain" or probably "penumbra is brain" for stroke patients is illustrated and consequently clinical evaluation, as well as technological studies are speeded-up, rather than traditional neurological examinations, a short but sufficient and therapy-related rather than diagnosis restricted repertoire is essential and includes all aspects of respiratory and cardiovascular function as well as scores of the level of consciousness (using the Glasgow Coma Scale, Fig. 1) and neurological and behavioral deficits (using the National Institutes of Health Stroke Scale, Fig. 2). Detailed investigation should be avoided, but medical and surgical history from patients and their relatives still are to be carefully considered with regard to previous stroke events, treatments for other cardiovascular diseases, etc.

Standard technical tests include:

(i) ECG
(ii) chest X-ray
(iii) blood sample studies/blood cell counts (including thrombocytes) glucose, creatinine, creatinin kinase or troponin, electrolytes, INR, APTT and toxic substance quinine.

An ECG should also be carried out because of the high incidence of heart conditions in this population. Stroke and myocardial infarction may occur

Glasgow Coma Scale			
	Best eye response	**Best verbal response**	**Best motor response**
5	—	Oriented	Obeys commands
4	Eyes open spontaneously	Confused	Localising pain
3	Eye opening on command	Inappropriate words	Withdrawal from pain
2	Eye opening to pain	Incomprehensible sounds	Extension to pain
1	No eye opening	No verbal response	No motor response
The GCS is scored between 3 (worst) and 15 (best) by adding the scores relating to each of three parameters: a score of ≥ 13 = mild brain injury, 9∝12 = moderate injury, ″ 8 = severe brain injury			

Glasgow Coma Scale

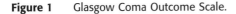

Glasgow Coma Scale	
Category	**Outcome**
1	Good recovery; independent lifestyle
2	Moderate disability; independent lifestyle
3	Severe disability; conscious but not independent
4	Vegetative state
5	Death

Figure 1   Glasgow Coma Outcome Scale.

together. Arrhythmias are frequently either the cause or the result of embolic stroke. Echocardiography should also be performed in most patients with stroke to document any cardioembolic source (thrombus in the left atrium or atrial septal aneurysm) or an atheroma in the arch of the aorta. Equally, an echocardiogram is necessary to detect a shunt of blood from the right to the left atrium through a patent foramen ovale or atrial septal defect. The accuracy of this ultrasound examination is greatly increased by transesophageal echocardiography and transcranial Doppler studies.

In the acute situation a separation between TIA and stroke is impossible and should not be accepted any longer not least as both prognosis and course of the disease are similar.

The same diagnostic studies are used for all patients with *brain attacks* whether ischemic or hemorrhagic are suspected: both groups need CT/MRI neuroimaging of the brain and vascular imaging including full cardiological work-up (Figs. 3 and 4).

CCT is the method of choice in both the acute and follow-up evaluation of cerebrovascular diseases, since its introduction in the early 1970s. Advantages of

NIH Stroke Scale

Assess level of consciousness

Alert	0
Drowsy	1
Stupourous	2
Coma	3

Assess orientation (month, age)

Both correctly	0
One correctly	1
Two incorrect	2

Follow commands
(1. Open and close eyes
2. Make fist and release)

Obeys both correctly	0
Obeys one correctly	1
Two incorrect	2

Follow my finger

Normal	0
Partial gaze palsy	1
Forced deviation	2

Visual field

Normal	0
Partial hemianopia	1
Complete hemianopia	2
Bilateral loss	3

Facial palsy
(Show teeth, raise eyebrows, squeeze eyes shut)

Alert	0
Drowsy	1
Stupourous	2
Coma	3

Motor strength for each of 4 limbs
(Passively move extremity and observe strength)
a. Elevate left arm to 90 degrees
b. Elevate right arm to 90 degrees
c. Elevate left leg to 30 degrees
d. Elevate right leg to 30 degrees

No drift	0
Drift	1
Some effort against gravity	2
No effort against gravity	3
No movement	4
Amputation, joint fusion (untestable)	9

Co-ordination of limb ataxia

Absent	0
Present in upper or lower	1
Present in both	2

Sensory
(1. Pin prick to face, arm, trunk and legs
2. Compare sides)

Normal	0
Partial loss	1
Dense loss	2

Speech clarity while reading word list

Normal articulation	0
Mild-moderate slurring	1
Nearly unintelligible, mute	2
Intubated or other physical barrier	3

Language (Describe picture, name items, read sentences)

No aphasia	0
Mild-moderate aphasia	1
Severe aphasia	2
Mute	3

Extinction and inattention

No neglect	0
Partial neglect	1
Profound neglect	2

Total

Figure 2   National Institute of Health Stroke Scale.

magnetic resonance imaging (MRI) are: excellent tissue contrast, high sensitivity for detecting early ischaemic and high susceptibility for demonstration of even very small haemorrhagic findings. Detection of flow parameters are excellent, although delineation of acute and developing penumbra surrounding the ischemic core or

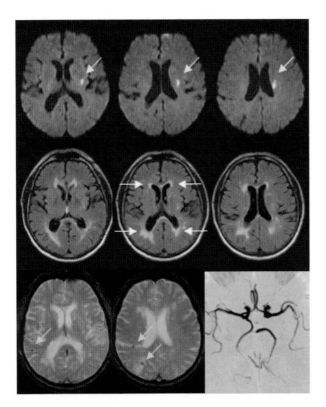

Figure 3   Typical MRI findings in a 78-year-old stroke patient with cerebral microangiopathy. Diffusion-weighted images (upper row) show a single hyperintense acute ischemic lesion in the territory of a perforating artery (arrow). The T_2-weighted FLAIR technique (middle row) demonstrates quite extensive chronic white matter lesions in a pattern typical for subcortical vascular encephalopathy with hyperintense lesions in the para- and periventricular white matter. T_2^* susceptibility-weighted sequences (bottom left and middle) show several small cortical/subcortical microbleeds, while the MR angiography (bottom right) demonstrates irregular contrast of intracranial vessels – a finding suggesting arteriosclerosis.

infarction are still insufficient as are sometimes developing ischemic territories close to parenchymal hemorrhage. Already approved early specific stroke treatment with tPA requires CT within a short 3 h time frame, potentially beneficial but not scientifically evaluated (or additional when using other drugs, including combinations of new protective and thrombolytic agents). Beyond this time limit, successful treatment can only be established if MRI or specific CT methodologies are used facilitating separation of perfusion deficits surrounding the core of already developing tissue necrosis (i.e., an equivalent of the ischemic penumbra).

Conventional angiography first performed in 1927, today is only selectively used in acute stroke patients, but is still considered for early interventional

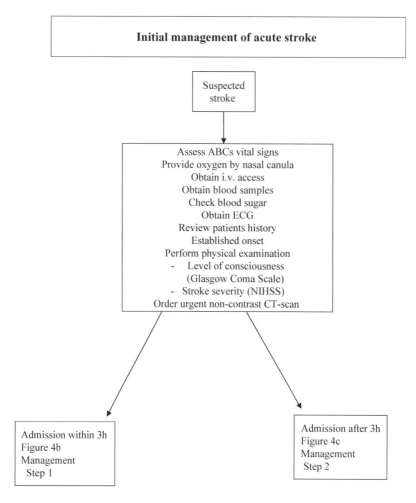

Figure 4a   Initial management of acute stroke.

treatment. Despite encouraging and evidence-based results of intra-arterial thrombolysis in the carotid system in RCTs, indications for angiography are left to patients with basilar artery thrombosis and suspected vascular malformations and bleeding aneurysms. They either need immediate treatment during the diagnostic procedure itself or after previous MRA/CTA/ultrasound studies have suggested interventional rather than surgical conservative therapy planning. MRA and modern ultrasonography have overtaken large domains of catheter angiography and further technical and software development for refined analysis and online investigation will demonstrate preferential use and utility of such techniques in early stroke monitoring. In addition, treatment perspectives using MR/ultrasound technologies are on the horizon and have been studied already

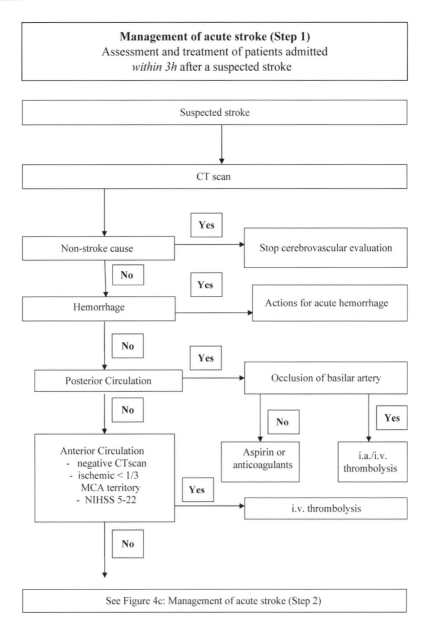

Management of acute stroke (Step 1)
Assessment and treatment of patients admitted
within 3h after a suspected stroke

Suspected stroke

CT scan

Non-stroke cause — **Yes** → Stop cerebrovascular evaluation

No

Hemorrhage — **Yes** → Actions for acute hemorrhage

No

Posterior Circulation — **Yes** → Occlusion of basilar artery

No   **No**   **Yes**

Anterior Circulation
- negative CTscan
- ischemic < 1/3
  MCA territory
- NIHSS 5-22

Aspirin or anticoagulants   i.a./i.v. thrombolysis

Yes → i.v. thrombolysis

No

See Figure 4c: Management of acute stroke (Step 2)

Figure 4b   Management of acute stroke (Step 1).

in clinical trials. However, in patients with hemorrhagic strokes and subarachnoid hemorrhage that form 15%–20% of all stroke cases, conventional angiography will continue to represent the gold standard for diagnosis and increasingly for therapeutic interventions (e.g., coiling of aneurysms) as well or beyond neurosurgery.

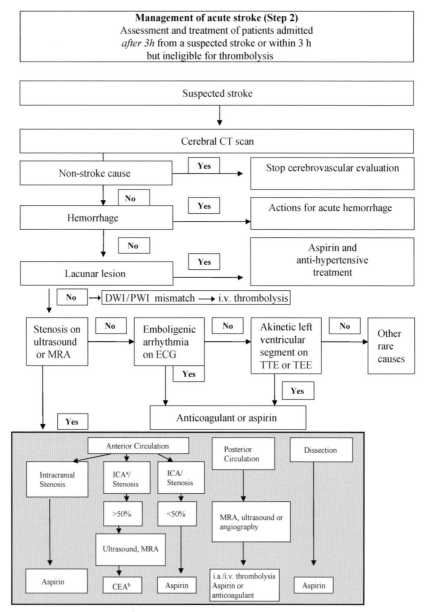

Figure 4c   Management of acute stroke (Step 2).

The rapid development of non-invasive ultrasound techniques has resulted in a broad array of clinical applications for the assessment of both extracranial and intracranial arterial diseases, both in the acute and chronic conditions. Rather than providing information for the diagnosis and staging of various obstructive cerebrovascular diseases, the capacity of ultrasound to identify and monitor continuously (on the ICU and Stroke Unit) and conditions of cerebrovascular circulation and brain perfusion in three dimensions and is preferential as well as the new application for sonothrombolysis. In addition, administration of micro-bubble encapsulated agents and drugs to selected focal areas within the brain by external destruction of their carrier demonstrates the perspectives of these techniques in acute stroke management.

Because of the advances in morphologic and functional neuroimaging, the diagnostic utility of electrophysiologic investigations, such as electroencephalography, and EP recordings have been dropped, reduced or even abandoned. However, these techniques still offer excellent chances for monitoring of brain functions of patients treated for complications and prevention of further brain tissue deterioration for the analysis of mechanism underlying clinical symptoms discrepant from neuroimaging findings. In particular, for the prognosis of functional outcome, they seem to provide far more relevant information than considered at present along with the best temporary resolution available and low cost. Sensory and motor EPs also are helpful in understanding mechanisms of recovery and reorganization in stroke patients and are indeed the only methodology at present to support a reliable prognosis.

Cardiovascular investigations on site and in close cooperation within the Stroke Team taking care of acute stroke patients are important for three major reasons: *first*, cerebral injury may force cardiac damage, even in patients without pre-existing cardiac disease; *second*, brain attacks may be cardioembolic in about 20%–30% of the cases and *third*, more than one-half of vascular patients may have co-existing coronary artery disease and the risk of coronary events with long-term follow-up exceeds the risk of cerebrovascular recurrences. While the last two reasons are commonly well considered, the first is still debated: knowledge on the pathophysiology of the autonomic system and the increasing number of patients with cerebral death as a possible donor for heart transplantations suggest that the cardiac consequences of cerebral damage is by far underestimated. Electrocardiographic monitoring has identified numbers of life-threatening ventricular arrhythmias in stroke patients treated on Stroke Units with continuous ECG monitoring and consequent treatment has rescued many of them from acute formerly suspected "stroke death." Acute cerebral damage may cause myocardial damage which can be documented by two-dimensional echocardiography, serum markers and myocardial necrosis; the clinical relevance of this is uncertain at present. Possible triggers of ventricular arrhythmia are hypoglycemia, hypoxia, autonomic nervous system imbalance and q-t prolongation; some of them can be promptly identified and adequately treated.

Biologic System	Test	Compartment	Method	Significance	Current Clinical Value
Glucose metabolism	Glucose (fasting, tolerance) HbA1c	Blood, urine plasma	Hexokinase method chromatography	Vascular risk factor, Diagnostic	Routine
Lipid metabolism	Cholesterol, triglycerides HDL/LDL-cholesterol	Blood	Enzymatic and precipitation techniques	Vascular risk factor	Routine
	Lp (a)	Blood	ELISA	Vascular risk factor	Routine
Methionine metabolism	Homocyst(e)ine	Blood, urine	HPLC	Diagnostic	Selected conditions
Antithrombotic systems	AT III, protein C, protein S	Plasma	Chromogenic assays, coagulometry	Diagnostic	Selected conditions
Coagulation and fibrinolysis	Prothrombin time, aPTT	Blood	Coagulometry, photometry	Therapy monitoring	Routine
	FM, FpA, TAT, F1+2 D-dimer, B-β-peptide	Plasma	ELISA	Pathogenic	Selected conditions
Systemic host defence	ESR, WBC, CRP	Blood serum	Westergren, impedance counter method, nephelometry	Investigation of acute phase reaction	Routine
	IL-6, IL-1β, TNF-ᾶ sICAM-1, sELAM-1, sL-selectin	Serum Plasma	Nephelometry, ELISA ELISA	Endothelial activation	Selected conditions
Viscosity of blood	Hematocrit, fibrinogen	Blood	Microhematocrit technique, coagulometry	Risk factor, pathophysiologic	Routine
	Whole blood, plasma viscosity, cell aggregability	Plasma	Filtration technique, shear-viscosimeter, aggregometer		Experimental
HPA system	Cortisol, ACTH	Plasma	RIA	Pathophysiologic Prognostic	Experimental
Immune system	ANA, anti-dsDNA Sm-Ag, Scl-70, ANCA	Serum	Immunofluorescence, RIA	Diagnosis of vasculitis (e.g. SLE)	Selected conditions
	Lupus anticoagulant / anticardiolipin Ab's	Plasma	Coagulometry ELISA	Pathogenetic	Selected conditions
Brain tissue integrity	NSE, S-100 protein	Serum, CSF	RIA	Prognostic	Selected conditions

Figure 5   Synopsis of Biologic and Immunologic Tests on Cerebrovascular Diseases.

Sources of cardioembolic stroke, whether from coexisting cardiovascular or cardiac diseases need to be diagnosed early and treated immediately to improve late prognosis, because of the coexistence of cerebrovascular and cardiovascular diseases in almost every second patient. A brain attack can be considered a "warning sign" for future coronary events and therefore should be of utmost importance in the network of secondary prevention.

A lumbar puncture for cerebral spinal fluid analysis is not necessary in the regular patient who presents with cerebrovascular disease; however, it may be indicated if intracranial hemorrhages are suspected (parenchymal and subarachnoid hemorrhages as well as cerebral venous thrombosis) or if forms of isolated angitis or systemic vasculitis with CNS involvement are considered. Biomarkers indicating neuronal damage, inflammatory reactions, apoptosis, or poststroke reorganization tissue-associated activities (e.g., superoxide dismotase) are currently targets of scientific interest; however, whether taken from the CSF or from the blood, they so far have failed to directly influence diagnosis (ischemia vs hemorrhage separation) and therapeutic decisions (staging of acute stroke development within 72 hours). Only a small number of laboratory tests (Fig. 5) belong to the routine workup of stroke patients, a second group of tests is available to detect rare conditions, such as coagulation abnormalities, antiphospholipid syndromes, vasculitis and hyperviscosity syndromes in selected patients. A third very heterogeneous group of laboratory tests still awaits validation for its clinical usefulness, but at present is considered as experimental.

The history of George Frederick Handel's stroke may guide us on rehabilitation after stroke reminding us about the enormous capacity of brain plasticity. Once acute stroke treatment and monitoring on the Stroke Unit is terminated, continuous physiotherapy to improve functional reorganization may be necessary at least in some patients with good prognosis according to very recent but few fMRI and clinical studies, but often for reintegration in family and local social environment. This issue has not adequately been investigated scientifically despite huge amounts of money spent on rehabilitation compared to acute stroke treatment costs and secondary prevention measures.

Convalescence at the hot baths of Aachen brought George Frederick Handel a considerable improvement. "After a week he could drag himself along, after a second week he could move his arm and with enormous 'will power' and confidence, he tore himself out of the paralysis of death, for life to be much more fervent than before with every unutterable happiness, as only the recovered know. As "Hallelujah" boomed out for the first time, there was a great cheer . . . and this was raised again with the last "Amen," . . . the jubilation had scarcely filled the room with applause, he simply slipped away, not to thank the people who wanted to thank him, but rather the grace that had endowed this work."

Common cases of stroke

Dysarthria and clumsy hand syndrome

Clinical history

A 64-year-old man presented to our emergency room 12 hours after the sudden onset of slurring of his speech and incoordination of his right upper extremity. He reported that he was unable to write or to dial a phone number because of clumsiness of his fingers. Eight weeks before, he had noticed a transient, 30-minute lasting, hemisensory disturbance involving his left arm and leg.

General history

The patient was treated by his family physician for hypertension with a diuretic and with oral antidiabetics for his Type II diabetes.

Examination

On neurological examination he was dysarthric, had a mildly decreased nasolabial fold on the right and had a marked disturbance of diadochokinetic movements besides a mild paresis of his right upper extremity. Deep tendon reflexes were slightly increased on the right. There was no sensory disturbance, his gait was a bit unsteady.

Neurological scores on admission

NIH 4; Barthel Index 80; GCS 15.

Special studies

Cranial MRI revealed an acute small lacunar lesion in the internal capsule on the left besides several chronic white matter lesions in both hemispheres. In addition, multiple punctuate lesions, hypodense in T_1-weighted scans and hyperdense in T_2-weighted scans, were seen in the bilateral deep white matter that were interpreted as enlarged Virchow–Robin spaces. Transcranial magnetic stimulation and sensory evoked potentials were normal. No embolic source could be identified in transthoracic echocardiogram, ECG was normal with a normal sinus rhythm.

Serum analysis revealed an elevated Hemoglobin A1c with 6.9% and an elevated serum homocysteine (23.4 fmol/l).

Follow-up

The patient was transferred to a rehabilitation hospital 1 week after onset of symptoms. His medication on discharge included aspirin 100 mg/day, triamterene and hydrochlorothiazide in fixed combination, and metformin.

Image findings

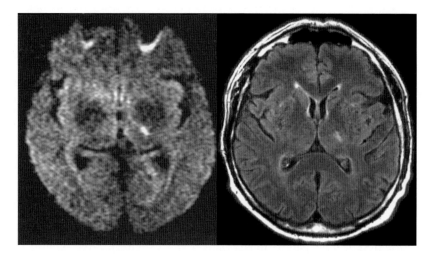

Figure 1.1   Diffusion-weighted MRI displaying a single acute lacunar lesion in the left internal capsule (*left*). The FLAIR scan shows no other pathology besides this single lesion (*right*).

Diagnosis

Dysarthria clumsy hand syndrome due to lacunar stroke in the posterior limb of the left internal capsule.

General remarks

Lacune is an old anatomical term that always has been discussed controversially. Historically, the first controversy arose regarding lacunes and other cavities in the brain. Later, the etiology of lacunes was debated in that some authors favored infarctions vs. hemorrhages vs. inflammatory changes. In the 1960s, C. Miller Fisher reported a large series of neuropathological studies in patients with lacunes and introduced several clinical syndromes on the basis of pathological findings. Even today, although enhanced through recent developments in neuroimaging, the lacunar concept, i.e., occlusion of a single penetrating artery leading to infarction in the depending territory is still debatable as other pathomechanisms can mimic the same clinical and neuroimaging patterns (e.g. Case 54). Besides increasing age, associated risk factors are most importantly arterial hypertension, especially at night-time, followed by diabetes and hyperhomocysteinemia. The long-term prognosis after a first lacunar infarction has been traditionally regarded as favorable; however, more recent prospective studies have shown, that in the long term, the risk of death is increased, mainly from cardiovascular disease. Moreover, since diffuse progressive white matter changes are often associated with (recurrent) lacunar stroke, the syndrome of subcortical vascular encephalopathy, SVE (syn. subcortical ischemic vascular disease) may develop, which leads to progressive cognitive and functional decline with a progressive dysexecutive syndrome and gait unsteadiness as the cornerstones of the disease.

Miller-Fisher described a series of more than 20 distinct lacunar syndromes. At least the first four of this series have become general neurological knowledge: (1) pure sensory stroke, (2) pure motor hemiparesis, (3) ataxic hemiparesis, (4) dysarthria-clumsy hand syndrome. The latter syndrome has been associated with a lesion in the basis pontis in the single pathological correlation in Fisher's first description. Later clinico-anatomical studies found that "internal capsule and pons are the most frequent cerebral sites."

FIRST DESCRIPTION

Durand-Fardel, M. *Traité du ramolissement du cerveau*. Paris: Baillère, 1843.

Marie, P. Des foyers lacunaires de désintégration et de différents autres états cavitaires du cerveau. *Rev. Méd.* (Paris) 1901; **21**:281.

CURRENT REVIEW

Norrving, B. Long-term prognosis after lacunar infarction. *Lancet Neurol.* 2003; **2**:238–245.

SUGGESTED READING

Arboix, A., Bell, Y., Garcia-Eroles, L. *et al.* Clinical study of 35 patients with dysarthria-clumsy hand syndrome. *J. Neurol. Neurosurg. Psychiatry* 2004; **75**:231–234.

Besson, G., Hommel, M., & Perret, J. Risk factors for lacunar infarcts. *Cerebrovasc. Dis.* 2000; **10**:387–390.

Fisher, C. M. Lacunes: small, deep cerebral infarcts. *Neurology* 1965; **15**:774–784.

Fisher, C. M. Pure sensory stroke involving face, arm, and leg. *Neurology* 1965; **15**:76–80.

Fisher, C. M. A lacunar stroke. The dysarthria-clumsy hand syndrome. *Neurology* 1967; **17**:614–617.

Fisher, C. M. The arterial lesions underlying lacunes. *Acta Neuropathol.* (Berl.) 1968; **12**:1–15.

Fisher, C. M. Ataxic hemiparesis. A pathologic study. *Arch. Neurol.* 1978; **35**:126–128.

Fisher, C. M. Lacunar strokes and infarcts: a review. *Neurology* 1982; **32**:871–876.

Fisher, C. M. & Cole, M. Homolateral ataxia and crural paresis: a vascular syndrome. *J. Neurol. Neurosurg. Psychiatry* 1965; **28**:48–55.

Glass, J. D., Levey, A. I., & Rothstein, J. D. The dysarthria-clumsy hand syndrome: a distinct clinical entity related to pontine infarction. *Ann. Neurol.* 1990; **27**:487–494.

Schonewille, W. J., Tuhrim, S., Singer, M. B., & Atlas, S. W. Diffusion-weighted MRI in acute lacunar syndromes. A clinical–radiological correlation study. *Stroke* 1999; **30**:2066–2069.

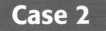

Sudden numbness of the right extremities

Clinical history

An 80-year-old woman came to the emergency room 24 hours after suddenly noticing a "strange" sensations in her right body. She noticed numbness and tingling in her right upper and lower extremities, trunk, and in the right half of her face. When trying to get up and walk, she noticed very mild unsteadiness and she recognized that her hand coordination was less precise.

General history

The patient was treated by her primary care physician for hypertension and slight hyperlipidemia. She reported chronic back pain due to osteodegenerative disease.

Examination

She had a hemisensory syndrome involving the face, trunk, and upper and lower limbs with predominant paresthesias and numbness. On motor examination, she showed very slight incoordination of the right hand, her gait was a bit unsteady and small-stepped. The rest of her medical and neurological examinations were normal.

Neurological scores on admission

NIH 2; Barthel Index 100; GCS 15.

Special studies

Laboratory data were significant for a leukocytosis (12 000 cells/mm^3), an elevated C-reactive protein of 32 mg/l. Initial CT scan was negative. Ultrasound examination of the extra- and intracranial arteries showed slight arteriosclerotic vessel wall abnormalities but no stenosis. MRI using diffusion weighted imaging showed a small inferolateral thalamic lesion on the left, T$_2$-weighted and FLAIR scans demonstrated moderate periventricular white matter lesions.

Follow-up

The patient was discharged 5 days after the onset of symptoms, with a residual hemisensory syndrome. Four weeks later, she visited her family doctor because of a progressively unpleasant feeling in her right arm and leg. This was interpreted as caused by a thalamic pain syndrome and the unpleasant feelings responded fairly well to treatment with gabapentin 1600 mg/day.

Image findings

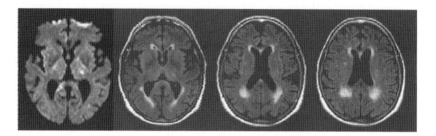

Figure 2.1 Diffusion-weighted MRI shows an acute inferolateral thalamic lesion on the left (*left image*), while T$_2$-weighted FLAIR sequences show symmetrical hyperintense lesions of the periventricular white matter due to cerebral microangiopathy.

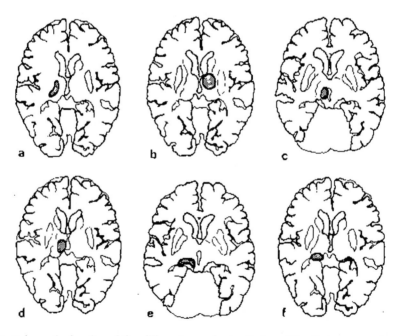

Figure 2.2 Schematic drawing of the different vascular territories of the thalamus: territory of the (a) thalamogeniculate/inferolateral artery, (b) anterior thalamoperforate artery, (c)(d) posterior choroidal artery, and (e)(f) posterior thalamoperforate artery. (b) is the only anterior circulation depending vascular territory infarction (according to Bogousslavsky *et al.*, 1988).

Diagnosis

Left inferolateral thalamic infarction due to microangiopathy.

General remarks

Vascular lesions of the thalamus destroy thalamic nuclei in different combinations and produce behavioral and sensorimotor syndromes depending
on which nuclei are involved. The main blood supply for the thalamus comes
from the proximal segments of the PCA through the paramedian, the inferolateral, and the posterior choroidal arteries. The remaining parts receive their
supply from the posterior communicating artery through the polar arteries.
Four classical thalamic stroke territories are described: The most common
thalamic infarcts involve either the inferolateral (syn. thalamogeniculate) (1)
or the paramedian (syn. thalamoperforant) (2) territories, the latter often
involve the upper midbrain as well and may be bilateral. The third type is the
posterior choroidal infarct (3), which has been reported rarely, compared to
the third most common type of thalamic stroke, anterior (syn. polar or tuberothalamic) (4) thalamic infarcts. Three variant types have been recently
reported.

The main clinical features in inferolateral territory strokes are a hemisensory
syndrome on occasion accompanied by slight hemiataxia and by slight motor
weakness. During follow-up, patients may report sometimes severe "thalamic"
pain syndrome. In comparison to the remaining thalamic stroke types, clinically
relevant cognitive dysfunction occurs rarely. Paramedian thalamic infarctions
produce a classical triad consisting of an acute decrease of arousal (especially
in bilateral lesions), neuropsychological abnormalities with a dysexecutive
syndrome, on occasion with memory impairment and aphasia in left-sided
lesions, and abnormal vertical gaze. Posterior choroidal infarctions manifest
with visual field abnormalities, commonly accompanied by a variable hemisensory loss. Some patients develop movement disorders such as dystonia or
tremor, on occasion with a delay of weeks or months. Polar or tuberothalamic
strokes are characterized by neuropsychological symptoms with executive dysfunction, memory loss and altered arousal and orientation, impairments of learning and memory, and changes in personality. The stroke mechanisms in thalamic
strokes are heterogeneous, although the classic thalamic syndromes do have predominant etiologies: a major proportion of paramedian strokes are due to cardiac
embolism, whereas most of inferolateral, tuberothalamic, and posterior choroidal
strokes are most often caused by microangiopathic lesions.

FIRST DESCRIPTION

Dejerine, J. & Roussy, G. Le syndrome thalamique. *Rev. Neurol. (Paris)* 1906; **14**:521–532.

CURRENT REVIEW

Carrera, E., Michel, P., & Bogousslavsky, J. Anteromedian, central, and posterolateral infarcts of the thalamus. Three variant types. *Stroke* 2004; **35**:2826–2831.

Schmahmann, J. D. Vascular syndromes of the thalamus. *Stroke* 2003; **34**:2264–2278.

SUGGESTED READING

Bogousslavsky, J., Regli, F., & Assal, G. The syndrome of unilateral tuberothalamic artery territory infarction. *Stroke* 1986; **17**:434–441.

Bogousslavsky, J., Regli, F., & Uske, A. Thalamic infarcts: clinical syndromes, etiology, and prognosis. *Neurology* 1988; **38**:837–848.

Caplan, L. R., DeWitt, L. D., Pessin, M. S., Gorelick, P. B., & Adelman, L. S. Lateral thalamic infarcts. *Arch. Neurol.* 1988; **45**:959–964.

Georgiadis, A. L., Yamamoto, Y., Kwan, E. S., Pessin, M. S., & Caplan, L. R. Anatomy of sensory findings in patients with posterior cerebral artery territory infarction. *Arch. Neurol.* 1999; **56**:835–838.

Hennerici, M., Halsband, U., Kuwert, T. *et al.* PET and neuropsychology in thalamic infarction: evidence for associated cortical dysfunction. *Psychiatry Res.* 1989; **29**:363–365.

Marsault, C., Agid, Y., & Vidailhet, M. Clinical characteristics and topography of lesions in movement disorders due to thalamic lesions. *Neurology* 2001; **57**:1055–1066.

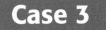

A 52-year-old woman with sudden hemiparesis

Clinical history

A 52-year-old woman was admitted to the stroke unit 5 hours after onset of a slight sensory–motor hemiparesis of the left extremities and a slight dysarthria accompanied by a dull right occipital headache. These symptoms improved within the first hour but persisted, and the patient reported that she had noticed similar symptoms 10 days earlier that had lasted less than an hour and had remitted completely.

General history

The patient weighed 119 kg with a body mass index of 43. She had had Type II diabetes for 10 years with symptoms of diabetic retinopathy and neuropathy. She was treated for hypertension and hypercholesterolemia.

Examination

On neurological examination she had a facial asymmetry and slight paresis of the left arm and leg as well as a paresthesia and numbness of the left side. Abnormal Babinski's reflex was present on the left.

Neurological scores on admission

NIH 6; Barthel Index 80; GCS 15.

Special studies

Ultrasound examination revealed an occlusion of the right ICA and a high grade (80%) stenosis of the left ICA. Transcranial Doppler showed collateral flow from the left to the right hemisphere via the anterior communicating artery and the posterior cerebral artery.

Follow-up

The patient was operated on the left ICA to restore cerebral perfusion and was treated with a platelet inhibitor (75 mg clopidogrel). In a follow-up examination 1 year later she was functioning well but still had a slight residual hemiparesis (NIH 3). She was independent in her daily activites (Barthel 95).

Image findings

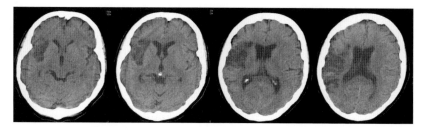

Figure 3.1   CT showed a territorial infarction in the right MCA territory from the insular/perisylvian to the parietal cortex, involving mainly the superior division of the MCA but sparing the lenticulostriate territory.

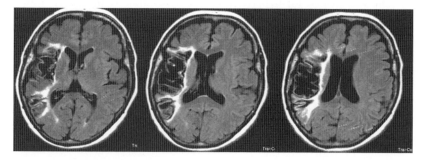

Figure 3.2   Follow-up MRI performed 1 year after the patient's stroke demonstrates a cystic lesion with atrophy and perilesional T_2-hyperintensity in the right MCA territory on FLAIR images.

Diagnosis

Territorial partial middle cerebral artery stroke.

General remarks

The infarct type in this patient is defined as a large ischemic lesion involving the cerebral cortex and subcortical structures in one or more major cerebral artery territories, referred to as "territorial infarction." The largest infarcts are those from proximal MCA occlusion, i.e. prelenticulostriate causing infarction in the basal ganglia, the adjacent capsular region, as well as extensive cortical territories. Occlusion of the proximal MCA can cause large territorial stroke with severe disability due to involvement of the internal capsule. The mechanism is embolism into or fresh thrombus in the intracranial arteries. The ACA territory may also be affected in some patients, and if the PCA arises from a fetal posterior communicating artery, an additional PCA stroke can occur. A partial MCA infarction occurs when the distal middle cerebral artery branch is occluded – if the occlusion is after the lenticulostriate vessels, the deep territory is spared. Occlusion of individual branches leads to restricted infarcts (M2 and M3 segments of the MCA).

Studies based on computed tomography have suggested that hemodynamically significant stenosis or obstructions of the extracranial ICA may cause hemodynamic changes in the distal regions of the hemispheric blood supply (ACA, MCA and/or PCA), the so-called border zones between major vascular territories, while embolism from ICA stenosis is believed to disproportionately affect the middle cerebral artery stem and distal branches producing territorial infarction, often including the lenticulostriate territory. In our series of 102 consecutive acute stroke patients with different degrees of ipsilateral ICA disease examined with diffusion-weighted MRI, we found territorial stroke in 47% of patients with ICA occlusion.

There is debate about whether it is appropriate to operate on a stenosed carotid artery after a recent brain infarct caused by a contralateral carotid artery occlusion such as this patient had. The left ICA in this case is probably asymptomatic but may be contributing to compromised collateral flow. During surgery which involves temporary occlusion of the artery, the infarct can grow. One of the editors (LRC) does not suggest operating on contralateral or distant arteries during the acute phase of brain ischemia but does suggest repair later. Other stroke experts do suggest more acute procedures as in this patient, in particular, if the patient's condition is unstable with early repeat TIAs.

FIRST DESCRIPTION

Fisher, C. M. Occlusion of the internal carotid artery. *Arch. Neurol. Psych.* 1951; **69**:346–377.

Fisher, C. M. Occlusion of the carotid arteries. *Arch. Neurol. Psych.* 1954; **72**:1876–1904.

SUGGESTED READING

Heinsius, T., Bogousslavsky, J., & Van Melle, G. Large infarcts in the middle cerebral artery territory. Etiology and outcome patterns. *Neurology* 1998; **50**:341–350.

Pessin, M. S., Hinton, R. C., Davis, K. R. *et al.* Mechanisms of acute carotid stroke. *Ann. Neurol.* 1979; **6**:245–252.

Szabo, K., Kern, R., Gass, A. *et al.* Acute stroke patterns in patients with internal carotid artery disease. *Stroke* 2001; **32**:1323–1329.

Rodda, R. A. & Path, F. R. C. The arterial patterns associated with internal carotid infarcts. *Stroke* 1986; **17**:69–75.

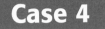

Sudden difficulty reading the left side of the morning paper

Clinical history

A 22-year-old man came to the emergency room because of sudden difficulty reading especially the left side of a newspaper, followed by severe right-side headache.

General history

His medical history was otherwise normal. He took no medication regularly, and had no known risk factors.

Examination

Neurological examination showed a nearly complete homonymous hemianopia with reduced optokinetic nystagmus but without other neuropsychological or sensorimotor deficits.

Neurological scores on admission

NIH 2; Barthel Index 100; GCS 15.

Special studies

Homonymous hemianopia was confirmed by Goldmann perimetry. Ultrasound examination of the extra- and intracranial vessels showed slightly reduced flow in the right posterior cerebral artery (30 cm/s maximal flow velocity) when compared with the left side (45 cm/s). A complete stroke evaluation including echocardiography and cardiac rhythm monitoring and testing for hematological disorders showed no abnormalities.

Follow-up

The visual field defect slightly improved during the first 2 weeks after symptom onset to a superior quadrantanopia. The patient was prescribed 100 mg aspirin daily for secondary prevention.

Image findings

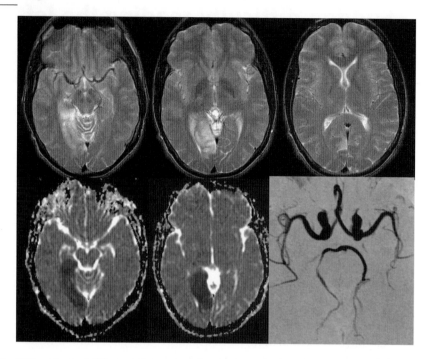

Figure 4.1   MRI performed 8 hours after onset of symptoms showed an acute ischemic lesion in the territory of the right PCA. The upper image row shows the edematous T_2-hyperintense lesion affecting the right optic radiation and in part the calcarine cortex. Maps of the apparent diffusion coefficient (ADC, *bottom row left and middle*) show signal reduction during the acute phase of the ischemia. The MRA shows reduced flow signal in the P_2-segment of the right PCA.

Diagnosis

Acute stroke in the posterior cerebral artery territory.

General remarks

Visual symptoms in stroke can either be visual perceptual abnormalities due to cerebral lesions or ocular symptoms caused by retinal disturbances. The nature of a visual field defect depends on the location of the lesion. The most common visual field defect caused by involvement of the striate cortex or the geniculo-calcarine tract is a homonymous hemianopia. Bilateral lesions cause bilateral hemianopic defects, often with sparing of portions of the visual fields. Some patients with cortical blindness deny visual difficulties and claim to see (Anton's syndrome). The second most common visual symptom in stroke patients is a temporary loss of vision in one eye, termed *transient monocular blindness* or *amaurosis fugax*. It can occur repeatedly in a stereotypic fashion during hours, days or weeks, each episode lasting seconds to minutes. Amaurosis fugax is regarded as a transient ischemic attack of the carotid artery territory caused by retinal emboli – typically reported in patients who have stenosis of the ipsilateral internal carotid artery. While in these patients imaging of the brain is often normal, cholesterol emboli (Hollenhorst plaques) can be detected in the branches of the central retinal artery by ophthalmoscopic examination.

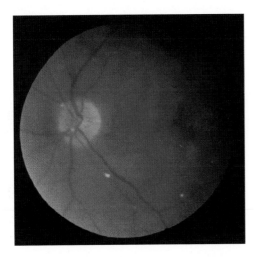

Figure 4.2 Ophthalmoscopic examination in a patient with recurrent transient monocular blindness due to a high grade stenosis of the ipsilateral internal carotid artery. Characteristic bright shiny bodies can be seen next to the branches of the central retinal artery.

FIRST DESCRIPTION

Hollenhorst, R. W. The ocular manifestations of internal carotid artery thrombosis. *Med. Clin. N. Am.* 1960; **44**:897–908.

Pessin, M. S., Lathi, E. S., Cohen, M. B. *et al.* Clinical features and mechanism of occipital infarction. *Ann. Neurol.* 1987; **21**:290–299.

SUGGESTED READING

Barton, J. S. & Caplan, L. R. Cerebral visual dysfunction. In Bogousslavsky, J. & Caplan, L. (eds.) *Stroke Syndromes*, 2nd edn. New York: Cambridge University Press, 2001; 87–110.

Caplan, L. R. Chapter 13. The posterior cerebral arteries. In Caplan, L. R. (ed.) *Posterior Circulation Disease. Clinical Findings, Diagnosis, and Management.* Cambridge MA: Blackwell Science, 1996; 444–491.

Caplan, L. R. Transient ischemia and brain and ocular infarction. In Albert, D. M., Jakobiec, F. A., Azar, D., & Gragoudas, E. (eds.) *Principles and Practice of Opthalmology,* 2nd edn. Philadelphia: W. B. Saunders Co, 2000; **5**:4224–4238.

Kumral, E., Bayulkem, G., Atac, C., & Alper, Y. Spectrum of superficial posterior cerebral artery territory infarcts. *Eur. J. Neurol.* 2004; **11**:237–246.

Wray, S. Visual symptoms (eye). In Bogousslavsky, J. & Caplan, L. (eds.) *Stroke Syndromes,* 2nd edn. New York: Cambridge University Press, 2001; 111–128.

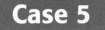

An 85-year-old man with difficulty expressing himself on the telephone

Clinical history

An 85-year-old man noticed difficulty expressing himself during a telephone conversation accompanied by a slight loss of strength in the right arm. He was brought to the emergency room within 1 hour; during this time his symptoms had nearly completely resolved.

General history

Arterial hypertension, hyperlipidemia, history of severe cardiac disease with myocardial infarction 6 years earlier, bradyarrhythmia, and reduced left-ventricular function.

Examination

The neurological examination showed slight amnestic aphasia with word-finding abnormalities.

Neurological scores on admission

NIH 1; Barthel Index 100; GCS 15.

Special studies

24-hour ECG recording showed intermittent atrial fibrillation and bradyarrhythmia with a mean heart rate of 53/min and pauses >5 seconds. Transthoracic echocardiography showed reduced left-ventricular function. Duplex sonography of the extracranial ICA diagnosed bilateral moderate (60%) proximal stenosis of the ICA.

Follow-up

The patient was referred to the cardiology department for the implantation of a permanent pacemaker and was treated with warfarin.

Image findings

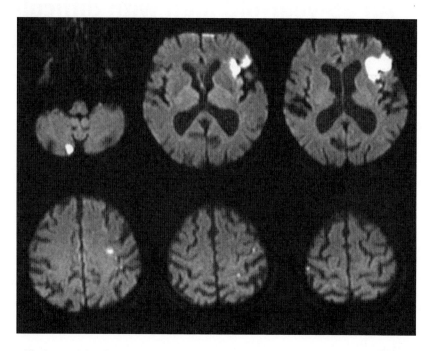

Figure 5.1   Diffusion-weighted MRI performed 8 hours after onset of symptoms showed not only the clinically suspected lesion in the superior division of the left anterior MCA territory associated with the patient's aphasia, but also an acute ischemic lesion in the right cerebellum and multiple punctuate lesions in cortical regions of both MCA territories associated with his motor dysfunction.

Diagnosis

Multiple brain infarcts in cardioembolic stroke.

General remarks

Only a small number of studies have addressed the issue of multiple brain infarcts in an attempt to correlate them with the underlying mechanisms and causes. In the CT-based patient population of the Lausanne Stroke Registry 3% had infarcts in multiple territories supplied by the carotid arteries, 2% had multiple infarcts in the vertebrobasilar artery territory, and 2% had multiple infarcts involving the territories of the carotid and vertebrobasilar arteries. In a more recent study of 329 consecutive ischemic stroke patients using diffusion weighted MRI acute multiple brain infarcts were detected in 28.9%. Well-recognized causes of multiple brain infarctions are atherosclerosis, emboligenic heart disease, and small vessel disease. Less frequent causes include inflammatory or non-inflammatory angiopathies, hematological disorders, hypoperfusion of the brain and venous infarcts, and malignancy-associated hypercoagulable states.

Special remarks

Cardioembolism causes approximately 20% of all ischemic strokes. The most frequent causes of cardioembolic stroke are non-rheumatic (often called non-valvular) atrial fibrillation, myocardial infarction, prosthetic valves, rheumatic heart disease, and ischemic cardiomyopathy. Atrial fibrillation is the most common cause of brain embolism. Patients with atrial fibrillation have an average annual risk of stroke of 2–15%. The risk varies according to the presence of certain risk factors, including older age, hypertension, poor left ventricular function, prior cardioembolism, diabetes, and thyrotoxicosis. Patients younger than 60 with none of these risk factors have an annual risk for stroke of about 0.5%, while those with most of the factors have a rate of about 15%. Guidelines for the use of warfarin are based on risk factors for brain embolism.

FIRST DESCRIPTION

Bogousslavsky, J. Double infarction in one cerebral hemisphere. *Ann. Neurol.* 1991; **30**:12–18.

Fisher, C. M. Reducing risks of cerebral embolism. *Geriatrics* 1979; **34**:59–66.

Wolf, P. A., Dawber, T. R., Thomas, H. E., & Kannel, W. B. Epidemiologic assessment of chronic atrial fibrillation and risk of stroke: The Framingham Study. *Neurology* 1978; **28**:973–977.

CURRENT REVIEW

Roh, J. K., Kang, D. W., Lee, S. H., Yoon, B. W., & Chang, K. H. Significance of acute multiple brain infarction on diffusion-weighted imaging. *Stroke* 2000; **31**:688–694.

SUGGESTED READING

Altieri, M., Metz, R. J., Müller, C., Maeder, P., Meuli, R., & Bogousslavsky, J. Multiple brain infarcts: clinical and neuroimaging patterns using diffusion-weighted magnetic resonance. *Eur. Neurol.* 1999; **42**:76–82.

Bogousslavsky, J., Bernasconi, A., & Kumral, E. Acute multiple infarction involving the anterior circulation. *Arch. Neurol.* 1996; **53**:50–57.

Caplan, L. R. Brain embolism. In Caplan, L. R., Hurst, J. W., & Chimowitz, M. I. (eds.). *Clinical Neurocardiology*, New York: Marcel Dekker Inc., 1999; 35–185.

Cerebral Embolism Task Force. Cardiogenic brain embolism: the second report of the Cerebral Embolism Task Force. *Arch. Neurol.* 1989; **46**:727–743.

Roh, J. K., Kang, D. W., Lee, S. H., Yoon, B. W., & Chang, K. H. Significance of acute multiple brain infarction on diffusion-weighted imaging. *Stroke* 2000; **31**:688–694.

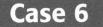

Case 6

Transient loss of vision

Clinical history

A 67-year-old man came to the hospital because of recurrent transient loss of vision in the left eye and sensorimotor hemiparesis of the right side. He had repeatedly had these symptoms during the previous 5 days, occurring for approximately 3–5 minutes and completely resolving. The transient visual loss appeared as a shade that descended over the left eye, usually clearing within 1 minute. The visual loss and right sided weakness occurred in different attacks, not together. However, on this particular day the paresis of the right side had lasted for almost 30 minutes.

General history

Arterial hypertension, cigarette smoking (20-pack–years), hyperlipidemia; no previous neurological symptoms.

Examination

Neurological examination revealed a slight drift of the extended extremities on the right side after 5 seconds and slightly increased tendon reflexes on the right side.

Neurological scores on admission

NIH 2; Barthel Index 100; GCS 15.

Special studies

A high grade stenosis with a local stenosis grade of 80% of the left extracranial ICA was present on ultrasound with a maximum systolic peak velocity of 2.8 m/s.

Follow-up

This patient was successfully treated with thrombendarterectomy and was discharged without neurological deficits. He was prescribed secondary prophylaxis with 100 mg aspirin a day.

Image findings

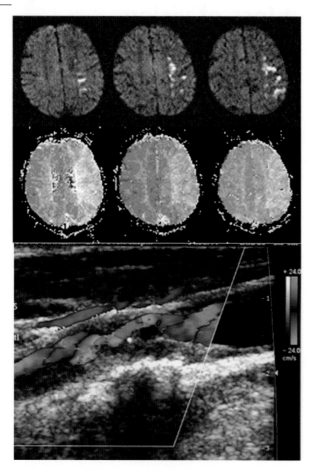

Figure 6.1   On diffusion-weighted MRI (*top*) small cortical and subcortical lesions are detected located mainly in hemodynamic risk zones. On perfusion-weighted maps (*middle*) hemodynamic compromise in the left middle cerebral artery territory is shown. Color-coded ultrasound image shows stenosis of the left ICA.

Diagnosis

Recurrent TIAs and hemodynamic stroke in a patient with severe left carotid artery stenosis.

General remarks

The stroke pattern of this patient, frequently termed "borderzone infarction," shows lesions predominantly located in one or more regions considered to be

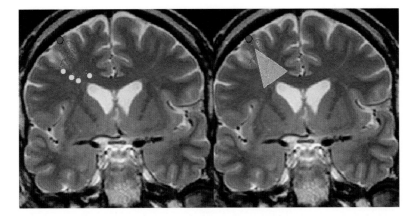

Figure 6.2   The theoretical concepts of stroke in hemodynamic risk zones – "dot-like" microembolic lesions in the most distal arterial branches resulting from more proximal vessel pathology and impaired emboli washout (*left*) and infarction of the compromised tissue in the borderzone territory (*right*).

hemodynamic risk zones between major cerebral vascular territories: the superficial or cortical border zones wedged between the anterior and middle cerebral artery, or between the middle and posterior cerebral artery, and the deep or subcortical border zone located in the vascular territory between deep and superficial arterial systems. Commonly, these lesions are small and dot-like or confluent distributed in a chain-like fashion and can be either single or multiple. These lesions have been described in patients with occlusive disease of the ICA and were believed to be caused by a gradual compromise of cerebral perfusion, especially under the conditions of limited collateral circulation. Modern concepts of hemodynamic lesions in patients with severe ICA stenosis emphasize the coexistence of hypoperfusion and arterial embolism.

Special remarks

Atherosclerotic narrowing of the ICA is a well-recognized cause of cerebral ischemia. The annual stroke risk for patients with symptomatic ICA stenosis is approximately 5% to 10%. In addition to a thorough ultrasound examination including transcranial Doppler or duplex to assess the patency and function of collateral pathways, a dedicated MRI protocol including diffusion-weighted as well as perfusion-weighted sequences should be performed in all patients with symptomatic ICA disease. The combination of DWI and PWI offers the possibility of identifying patients with potential to benefit from surgery or stenting.

In patients with recurrent TIAs due to high-grade stenosis, large perfusion deficits and a small acute ischemic lesion (the so-called DWI/PWI "mismatch"-constellation), early recanalization of the ICA should be achieved. Results from a recent study suggest that the recanalizing procedure should ideally be performed within a few weeks of the patient's last symptoms.

FIRST DESCRIPTION

Bogousslavsky, J. & Regli, F. Unilateral watershed cerebral infarcts. *Neurology* 1986; **36**:373–377.

Romanul, F. C. A. & Abramowicz, A. Changes in arterial borderzones. *Arch. Neurol.* 1964; **11**:40–65.

SUGGESTED READING

Caplan, L. R. & Hennerici, M. Impaired clearance of emboli (washout) is an important link between hypoperfusion, embolism, and ischemic stroke. *Arch. Neurol.* 1998; **55**:1475–1482.

Del Sette, M., Eliasziw, M., Streifler, J. Y. *et al.* Internal borderzone infarction: a marker for severe stenosis in patients with symptomatic internal carotid artery disease. *Stroke* 2000; **31**:631–636.

Johnston, S. C., Gress, D. R., Browner, W. S., & Sidney, S. Short-term prognosis after emergency department diagnosis of TIA. *J. Am. Med. Assoc.* 2000; **284**:2901–2906.

Rothwell, P. M., Eliasziw, M., Gutnikov, S. A., Warlow, C. P., & Barnett, H. J. Carotid Endarterectomy Trialists Collaboration. Endarterectomy for symptomatic carotid stenosis in relation to clinical subgroups and timing of surgery. *Lancet* 2004; **363**:915–924.

Szabo, K., Kern, R., Gass, A. *et al.* Acute stroke patterns in patients with internal carotid artery disease. *Stroke* 2001; **32**:1323–1329.

Waterston, J. A., Brown, M. M., Butler, P., & Swash, M. Small deep cerebral infarcts associated with occlusive internal carotid artery disease. A hemodynamic phenomenon? *Arch. Neurol.* 1990; **47**:953–957.

Massive intracerebral hemorrhage

Clinical history

A 64-year-old man, a heavy smoker with long-standing and poorly controlled arterial hypertension, was admitted with an acute left hemiparesis.

General history

Smoking (40-pack–years), arterial hypertension.

Examination

On the initial clinical evaluation, he was stuporous and hemiplegic on the left. The left pupil was slightly enlarged, but reactive to light. The blood pressure was 230/115 mmHg.

Neurological scores on admission

NIH 23; Barthel Index 0; GCS 5.

Special studies

Funduscopy revealed slight papilledema and chronic hypertensive changes. CT showed a large intracerebral hematoma in the right basal ganglia with intraventricular extension. The ventricles were already enlarged due to obstructive hydrocephalus.

Follow-up

After the patient deteriorated further and became comatose, surgical hematoma evacuation was performed 6 hours after the first onset of symptoms. In addition to the hematoma evacuation, an external ventricular drain was inserted. Initially, surgery was considered successful because the hematoma was nearly completely evacuated and the space-occupying effect, the cerebral blood flow and the hydrocephalus had normalized. However, clinically, the patient did not recover. He remained comatose and died a few weeks later from a prolonged respirator-associated pneumonia.

Image findings

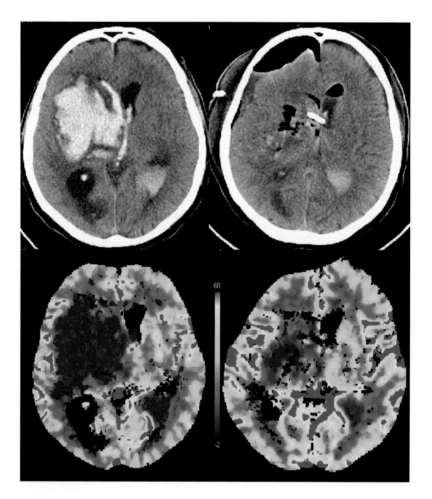

Figure 7.1 CT scan on admission (*top left*) shows a large, right-sided space-occupying hemorrhage originating from the basal ganglia with ventricular extension. The lateral ventricles are enlarged. The perfusion CT (*bottom left*) shows a marked reduction of the CBF in the entire right hemisphere. After evacuation of the hematoma and insertion of an external ventricular drain (*top right*), the space occupying effect was reduced and CBF normalized (*bottom right*).

Diagnosis

Spontaneous hypertensive intracerebral hemorrhage in the basal ganglia.

General remarks

Arterial hypertension is the most common cause of spontaneous ICH, accounting for about 60% of all cases. In the pathogenesis of hypertensive hemorrhages, degenerative processes within the arterial wall lead to lipohyalinosis and micro-aneurysms in the small perforating arteries. When a sudden increase of the cerebral blood flow happens, these vessels easily rupture. In many patients, intracerebral hemorrhage occurs near the time of onset of hypertension. The relatively abrupt rise in blood pressure causes rupture of arterioles unaccustomed to that level of hypertension.

Typically, hypertensive hemorrhages are located in the basal ganglia (caudate nucleus, putamen, internal capsule), thalamus, pons and the cerebellum. The small lenticulo-striate, thalamostriate, and pontine branches directly originate from large arteries, producing a massive pressure gradient. Nearly all patients with an acute ICH have a markedly elevated blood pressure. In those patients without history of arterial hypertension, it is not always possible to distinguish between previously undiagnosed hypertension or hypertension reactive to the ICH. Fun-duscopy may show chronic hypertensive changes in patients with undiagnosed arterial hypertension. However, arterial hypertension may be a cofactor in many patients with ICH due to other etiologies.

Special remarks

Rationale for surgical hematoma evacuation is the reduction of the intracranial mass effect to lower the acutely raised intracranial pressure. Protection of re-versibly damaged tissue in the surroundings of the hematoma is expected. Hematomas can be drained during open craniotomies or by a stereotactic approach in which the neurosurgeon introduces a catheter through a burr hole. Sometimes t-PA or another thrombolytic is introduced to liquify the hematoma to allow more complete evacuation – current RCTs are ongoing to investigate risk/benefit ratios.

The indications for hematoma evacuation in patients with supratentorial ICH are still unclear and controversial. Large randomized studies comparing medical and surgical treatment are scarce. The largest single study is still McKissock's carefully conducted trial dating back to 1961. A few subsequent smaller randomized trials and several uncontrolled studies yielded inconclusive results or were negative. A larger multicenter study (STICH), although weakened by some methodological flaws, also showed no benefit from surgery – unfortunately subgroup analysis was difficult and did not disclose any individual conditions. Considering the currently available data, the position, not to operate at all, is certainly justified, until the benefit of hematoma evacuation has been proven in a future study.

Future perspectives

A first clinical study has shown that activated recombinant coagulation factor VII (rFVIIa, NovoSeven®) can be administered safely to ICH patients and that rFVIIa given within 4 hours of onset can reduce the extent of hematoma growth in acute ICH.

CURRENT REVIEW

Broderick, J. P., Adams, H. P., Jr., Barsan, W. *et al.* Guidelines for the management of spontaneous intracerebral haemorrhage: A statement for healthcare professionals from a special writing group of the Stroke Council, American Heart Association. *Stroke* 1999; **30**:905–915.

SUGGESTED READING

Auer, L. M., Deinsberger, W., Niederkorn, K. *et al.* Endoscopic surgery versus medical treatment for spontaneous intracerebral hematoma: a randomized study. *J. Neurosurg.* 1989; **70**:530–535.

Batjer, H. H., Reisch, J. S., Allen, B. C., Plaizier, L. J., & Su, C. J. Failure of surgery to improve outcome in hypertensive putaminal hemorrhage. A prospective randomized trial. *Arch. Neurol.* 1990; **47**:1103–1106.

Davis, S. M., Broderick, J., Hennerici, M. *et al.* Recombinant Activated Factor VII Intracerebral Hemorrhage Trial Investigators. Hematoma growth is a determinant of mortality and poor outcome after intracerebral hemorrhage. *Neurology* 2006; **66**:1175–1181.

Fernandes, H. M., Gregson, B., Siddique, S., & Mendelow, A. D. Surgery in intracerebral hemorrhage. The uncertainty continues. *Stroke* 2000; **31**:2511–2516.

Hankey, G. J. & Hon, C. Surgery for primary intracerebral hemorrhage: is it safe and effective? A systematic review of case series and randomized trials. *Stroke* 1997; **28**:2126–2132.

Juvela, S., Heiskanen, O., Poranen, A. *et al.* The treatment of spontaneous intracerebral hemorrhage. A prospective randomized trial of surgical and conservative treatment. *J. Neurosurg.* 1989; **70**:755–758.

Mayer, S. A. Ultra-early hemostatic therapy for intracerebral hemorrhage. *Stroke* 2003; **34**:224–229.

Mayer, S. A., Brun, N. C., Begtrup, K. *et al.* Recombinant Activated Factor VII Intracerebral Hemorrhage Trial Investigators. Recombinant activated factor VII for acute intracerebral hemorrhage. *N. Engl. J. Med.* 2005; **352**:777–785.

McKissock, W., Richardson, A., & Taylor, J. Primary intracerebral haemorrhage: a controlled trial of surgical and conservative treatment in 180 unselected cases. *Lancet* 1961; **2**:221–226.

Case 8

Tinnitus during cycling in an orthopedic surgeon

Clinical history

A 40-year-old orthopedic surgeon came to the emergency room because of right-sided tinnitus. He had first noticed the tinnitus after his regular sunday bike-ride that consisted of 4 h hard cycling in mountainous terrain. He had no history of cardiovascular risk factors.

Examination

On examination he had an incomplete right Horner's syndrome (unilateral miosis and mild ptosis), but no further abnormalities. He had no headache, facial or neck pain or signs of cerebral ischemia. We heard no bruits when auscultating over the eyes and mastoids.

Neurological scores

NIH 0; Barthel Index 100; GCS 15.

Special studies

Cerebral CT, routine laboratory tests, and electrocardiography were all normal. Duplex ultrasound showed a normal lumen of both internal carotid arteries but a significant difference in flow signal. The right internal carotid artery had decreased flow-velocity and a hypopulsatile flow profile. This is a subtle, although undiagnostic, ultrasonographic evidence of a distal narrowing. Cerebral magnetic resonance angiography showed a right-sided carotid artery dissection with segmental loss of flow-signal and a hematoma in the ventral vessel wall. T_2 and diffusion-weighted magnetic resonance imaging showed no evidence of ischemia.

Follow-up

We prescribed aspirin to reduce the risk of embolization, and the tinnitus resolved completely within 1 week. The patient had no further symptoms.

Image findings

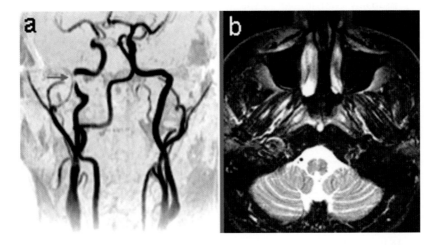

Figure 8.1   (a) Time-of-flight MRA with segmental loss of flow signal (arrow) in projection of the ICA siphon area. (b) T$_2$-weighted, transversal MRI with arrow indicating inhomogeneous structures of mural hematoma with dorsally located inner lumen of the right ICA.

Diagnosis

Dissection of the right internal carotid artery.

General remarks

While the overall incidence of spontaneous dissections of the extracranial vessels is 2.6 to 2.9 per 100 000, dissection of the ICA accounts for up to 20% of ischemic events in younger patients with a peak in the fifth decade, often in the absence of vascular risk factors. In contrast to traumatic arterial dissections, the term "spontaneous" refers to patients without severe trauma in temporal relationship to the dissection. Minimal neck torsion and "trivial traumata" such as coughing, sneezing, and normal sports activities are reported to precipitate carotid dissections in patients with an underlying structural abnormality of the arterial wall. Non-ischemic clinical features of arterial dissection, include (head–face–neck) pain, Horner's syndrome, tinnitus, and cranial nerve palsies.

Special remarks

Carotid artery dissection and traumatic plaque-rupture have been attributed to a variety of sporting activities. The proximity of the artery to the skull base probably accounts for dissections that occur in the absence of direct trauma. In this case, the cyclist's hyperextended neck, in combination with the rough terrain, probably contributed to the arterial dissection. Indeed, the ventral location of the hematoma is consistent with a ventral stretch on the vessel wall. The possibility of a carotid artery dissection should be considered in young patients presenting with acute onset of pulsatile tinnitus, Horner's syndrome or unusual severe head–face–neck pain.

CURRENT REVIEW

Schievink, W. I. Spontaneous dissection of the carotid and vertebral arteries. *N. Engl. J. Med.* 2001; **344**:898–906.

SUGGESTED READING

Hennerici, M., Steinke, W., & Rautenberg, W. High-resistance Doppler flow pattern in extracranial carotid dissection. *Arch. Neurol.* 1989; **46**:670–672.

Schievink, W. I., Mokri, B., & Piepgras, D. G. Spontaneous dissections of cervicocephalic arteries in childhood and adolescence. *Neurology* 1994; **44**:1607–1612.

Schievink, W. I., Mokri, B., & Whisnant, J. P. Internal carotid artery dissection in a community. Rochester, Minnesota, 1987–1992. *Stroke* 1993; **24**:1678–1680.

Steinke, W., Rautenberg, W., Schwartz, A., & Hennerici, M. Noninvasive monitoring of internal carotid artery dissection. *Stroke* 1994; **25**:998–1005.

Wiest, T., Hyrenbach, S., Bambul, P. *et al.* Genetic analysis of familial connective tissue alterations associated with cervical artery dissections suggests locus heterogeneity. *Stroke* 2006; **37**:1697–1702.

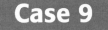

Case 9

Headache after an exhausting tennis match

Clinical history

A 55-year-old man developed a severe headache with acute exploding onset during the night. He recalled a stinging pain in the back of his head and vomiting after an exhausting tennis match 1 week before.

Examination

On admission, the patient did not have papilledema or focal neurological signs. He had persistent holocephalic headache but no fever, ear, or eye disease.

Neurological scores

NIH 0; Barthel Index 100; GCS 15.

Special studies

MRI scan of the brain showed a thrombus in the superior sagittal sinus and in the right transverse sinus without parenchymal hemorrhage or edema. Extensive screening for etiologically relevant factors did not show any abnormalities. There were no hematologic or inflammatory disorders or coagulopathy.

Follow-up

The patient was initially treated with low-molecular weight heparin. During the hospital stay, the headache improved after morphine was given; the patient was discharged with phenprocoumon (INR 2.0 to 2.5). At the 3-month follow-up examination the patient was free of symptoms accompanied by complete recanalization of the cerebral venous system on MRI. Therapy was replaced by a platelet function inhibitor (Clopidogrel 75 mg/d).

Image findings

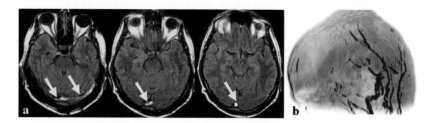

Figure 9.1 (a) Yellow arrows point to hyperintense signals along the course of the left transverse sinus and the superior sagittal sinus indicating thrombotic material which was also seen in the right transverse sinus to a lesser extent. (b) MR-venography shows lack of flow signal in both transverse sinuses and the superior sagittal sinus.

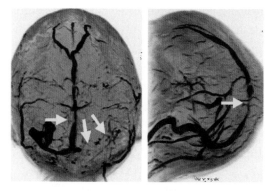

Figure 9.2 MR-venography after 3 months shows slight residual narrowing of the superior sagittal sinus (arrow), a partly recanalized left transverse sinus while the right side is completely recanalized (arrows).

Diagnosis

Cerebral sinus thrombosis.

General remarks

Cerebral sinus thrombosis is an uncommon cause of stroke. There is no exact data on the incidence, but since non-invasive diagnostic methods as CT and MRI of the cerebral venous system are now available, clinically inapparent or

Table 9.1. List of potential causes of cerebral venous thrombosis

Infectious	
Local	Otitis media
	Nasolabial and/or facial infections
	Pyogenic meningitis
Systemic	Septicemia *(e.g. gram negative)*
	Fungal infections
Non-infectious	
Focal	Compression of cerebral venous drainage by head or neck tumors
	Occlusion of the internal jugular vein
	Head injury
	Neurosurgical intervention
	After lumbar puncture, epidural, or spinal anesthesia
Systemic	General surgery
	Pregnancy and Puerperium
	Oral contraceptives
	Cardiac insufficiency
	Nephrotic syndrome
	Severe dehydration
	Malignancy *(lymphoma, leukemia)*
	Inherited thrombophilia *(e.g. Anti-thrombin III deficiency, Antiphospholipid Syndrome, Protein C & S alterations, Factor V Leiden and factor II gene mutations)*
	Acquired prothrombotic state
	Polycythemia vera and secondaria
	Thrombocythemia
	Anemia
	Hepatic cirrhosis, Crohn disease, ulcerative colitis
	Vasculitis
	Sarcoidosis
	Medications *(corticosteroids, L-asparaginase)*

moderate cases are being diagnosed. The long-term outcome is good. In a follow-up study of Preter *et al.*, 1996 with 77 patients, all survived and 86% had no remaining neurological deficit. In other studies the impairment-free outcome is around 80%. Mortality ranges below 10%. Common complications and deficits are persistent headache, seizures and in few patients neuropsychological dysfunction. Predictive factors for a poor outcome are impairment of consciousness, worsening of clinical symptoms, and deep venous drainage thrombosis.

Treatment remains controversial. The effect of heparin in the acute phase is not yet proven, however a number of studies conclude that the use of heparin decreases mortality – especially in more severe cases. Prophylactic therapy with long-term anticoagulation is also controversial. The recommendations are based upon the guidelines for peripheral deep vein thrombosis. The optimal duration of heparin is not established, but with the advent of neurologic improvement, heparin therapy is switched over to oral anticoagulation (warfarin) adjusted to maintain an INR between two and three.

Special remarks

Table 9.1 summarizes infectious and non-infectious settings known to be associated with cerebral venous thrombosis. Despite the continuing description of new causes, the proportion of cases with unknown etiology remains between 20% and 35% in a recent series. In our patient, the only potential factor was dehydration during an exhausting tennis match 1 week earlier. We recommend that these patients be followed over the next few years, as this might lead to the identification of an underlying cause, most often a systemic disease.

A negative D-dimer assay often supports the diagnosis of cerebral venous thrombosis and susceptibility-weighted MR images are of high diagnostic value in oligosymptomatic cases such as ours presuading only with headache.

FIRST DESCRIPTION

Barnett, H. J. M. & Hyland, H. H. Non-infective intracranial venous thrombosis. *Brain* 1953; **76**:36–49.

Garcin, R. & Pestel, M. *Thrombophlébites Cérébrales*. Paris: Masson et Cie, 1949.

Ribes, M. F. Des recherches faites sur la phlébite. *Rev. Méd. Française Etrangère et J. Clin. l'Hotel-Dieu Charité de Paris*. 1825; **3**:5–41.

CURRENT REVIEW

Crassard, I. & Bousser, M. G. Cerebral venous thrombosis. *J. Neuroophthalmol.* 2004; **24**:156–163.

SUGGESTED READING

Bousser, M.-G. Antithrombotic strategy in stroke. *Thromb. Haemost.* 2001; **86**:1–7.

Bousser, M.-G. & Ross-Russell, R. *Cerebral Venous Thrombosis*. London: W. B. Saunders, 1997.

Crawford, S. C., Digre, K. B., Palmer, C. A., Bell, D. A., & Osborn, A. G. Thrombosis of the deep venous drainage of the brain in adults. Analysis of seven cases with review of the literature. *Arch. Neurol.* 1995; **52**:1101–1108.

Cumurciuc, R., Crassard, I., Sarov, M., Valade, D., & Bousser, M. G. Headache as the only neurological sign of cerebral venous thrombosis: a series of 17 cases. *J. Neurol. Neurosurg. Psychiatry* 2005; **76**:1084–1087.

De Bruijn, S. F., de Haan, R. J., & Stam, J. For the Cerebral Venous Sinus Thrombosis Study Group. Clinical features and prognostic factors of cerebral venous sinus thrombosis in a prospective series of 59 patients. *J. Neurol. Neurosurg. Psychiatry* 2001; **70**:105–108.

De Bruijn, S. F. & Stam, J. Randomized, placebo-controlled trial of antocoagulant treatment with low-molecular-weight heparin for cerebral sinus thrombosis. *Stroke* 1999; **30**:484–488.

Idbaih, A., Boukobza, M., Crassard, I., Porcher, R., Bousser, M. G., & Chabriat, H. MRI of clot in cerebral venous thrombosis: high diagnostic value of susceptibility-weighted images. *Stroke* 2006; **37**:991–995.

Kuehnen, J., Schwartz A., Neff, W., & Hennerici, M. Cranial nerve syndrome in thrombosis of the transverse / sigmoid sinuses. *Brain* 1998; **121**:381–388.

Preter, M., Tzourio, C., Ameri, A., & Bousser, M. G. Long-term prognosis in cerebral venous thrombosis. Follow-up of 77 patients. *Stroke* 1996; **27**:243–246.

Wetzel, S. G., Kirsch, E., Stock, K. W., Kolbe, M., Kaim, A., & Radue, E. W. (1999) Cerebral veins: comparative study of CT-venography with intraarterial digital subtraction angiography. *Am. J. Neuroradiol.* 1999; **20**:249–255.

Case 10

Anticoagulation-associated hemorrhage

Clinical history

A 52-year-old man was admitted with aphasia and right hemiparesis of sudden onset. The patient had an artificial aortic valve after an infectious endocarditis 12 years ago. Since that time, he had been treated with warfarin.

Examination

On the initial clinical evaluation, he was aphasic and had a moderate right-sided hemiparesis.

Special studies

The INR on admission was 2,9, well within the target boundaries. Immediately after the diagnosis was established, he was treated with fresh plasma concentrates to halt the hematoma expansion. Transesophageal echocardiography revealed no unexpected findings. After 24 hours, anticoagulation was continued with unfractioned heparin (target PTT 60s). Over the next few days, the patient gradually deteriorated and transiently developed a complete hemiplegia. In repeated follow-up CTs, the hematoma size remained unchanged but a marked perifocal edema developed, which gradually disappeared over the next 2 weeks. Correspondingly, the patient's symptoms improved.

Follow-up

One month after the hemorrhage, he still had a residual hemiparesis and moderate aphasia, but was able to walk without aid.

Image findings

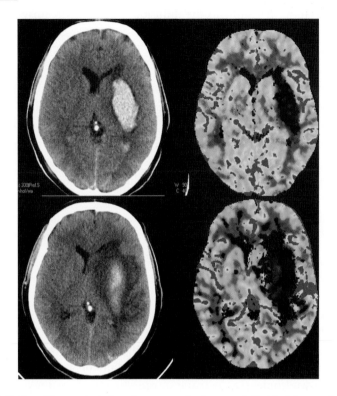

Figure 10.1 The CT on admission (*upper row*) shows a left-sided hemorrhage in the basal ganglia without ventricular extension. The space-occupying effect is moderate. With the perfusion CT (*right*), the CBF is reduced in the region of the hemorrhage only. Eight days later (*lower row*), a marked perifocal edema has developed with a large zone of a reduced CBF surrounding the hematoma.

Diagnosis

Intracerebral hemorrhage under anticoagulant therapy with perifocal edema.

General remarks

About 10% of all ICHs are caused by coagulation disorders, in most cases after anticoagulant treatment with warfarin or heparin. In a large study sample of 3862 patients with long-term anticoagulation, 1.6% developed ICH. Additional risk factors for ICH such as arterial hypertension or subcortical vascular encephalopathy, which may predispose for ICH, are frequently present in this patient group. However, the hemorrhage may well be in a location typical for hypertensive hemorrhages. In some patients, it remains unclear whether the hemorrhage was the primary event or secondary to an embolic ischemic infarction. Demonstration of lesions in the diffusion-weighted MR images may help to distinguish these etiologies. However, in most situations, this question is of no therapeutic relevance. Typical features of ICH in patients with coagulation disorders are a large hematoma volume and a high mortality.

After systemic fibrinolytic therapy of myocardial infarction, the frequency of ICH is below 1%. However, after systemic fibrinolysis for cerebral infarction, the risk for parenchymatous hemorrhage is increased (2%–4%). Moreover, the risk of hemorrhagic transformation or symptomatic parenchymatous hemorrhage within the area of an ischemic infarct is increased under a therapy with heparin of any type. In patients with an absolute indication for anticoagulant therapy such as an artificial heart valve, the risk of ICH enlargement has to be weighted against the risk of thrombosis of the valve. In those patients, the minimum possible dose of heparin is given in the acute phase of the disease.

Special remarks

In the acute phase, the hemorrhage itself is the main contributor for the space-occupying effect. During the following days, secondary effects such as hydrocephalus and perifocal brain edema may greatly augment the space-occupying effect, leading to dislocation and compression of more distant parts of the brain and herniation syndromes. In the tissue surrounding the hematoma, mechanical compression and the release of vasoconstrictive substances from the hematoma cause a marginal zone of complete ischemia, followed by an area of relative ischemia which is comparable to the penumbra in ischemic infarction. However, the exact mechanisms that lead to the perifocal edema in intracerebral hemorrhage are not well elucidated yet and are an issue of debate; there are also studies that have not demonstrated a zone of perifocal ischemia. It is of importance that the area of the perifocal edema may exceed the hematoma size. This mechanism is the cause of a frequently observed transient clinical deterioration during the first days after ICH, e.g., a transient aphasia in patients with basal ganglia hemorrhage. The perifocal ischemia leads to a perifocal cytotoxic brain edema within 24 to 48 hours after the ictus, typically increasing over several days and may lead to a delayed rise in the intracranial pressure. In addition to ischemia, several other mechanisms such as inflammatory responses, the release of toxic substances from the degrading hematoma, excitatory transmitters, and leukotrienes contribute to the perifocal brain edema. These mechanisms could be target points for therapies with immunosuppressive or neuroprotective drugs in the future (Lees *et al.*, 2006). Up to now, there is no established therapy for the post-hemorrhagic brain edema. Corticosteroids are not effective, and the use of osmotic agents is questionable.

CURRENT GUIDELINE

Broderick, J. P., Adams, H. P., Jr., Barsan, W. *et al.* Guidelines for the management of spontaneous intracerebral hemorrhage: a statement for healthcare professionals from a special writing group of the Stroke Council, American Heart Association. *Stroke* 1999; **30**:905–915.

SUGGESTED READING

Brott, T., Broderick, J., Kothari, R. *et al.* Early hemorrhage growth in patients with intracerebral hemorrhage. *Stroke* 1997; **28**:1–5.

Caplan, L. R. General symptoms and Signs. In Kase, C. S. & Caplan, L. R. (eds.) *Intracerebral Hemorrhage.* Boston, MA: Butterworth-Heinemann 1994; 31–43.

Coon, W. W. & Willis, P. W. Hemorrhagic complications of anticoagulant therapy. *Arch. Intern. Med.* 1974; **133**:386–392.

Eckman, M. H., Rosand, J., Knudsen, K. A., Singer, D. E., & Greenberg, S. M. Can patients be anticoagulated after intracerebral hemorrhage? *Stroke* 2003; **34**:1710–1716.

Gebel, J. M., Jauch, E. C., Brott, T. G., Khoury, J., Sauerbeck, L., Salisbury, S., Spilker, J., Tomsick, T. A., Duldner, J., & Broderick, J. P. Natural history of perihematomal edema in patients with hyperacute spontaneous intracerebral hemorrhage. *Stroke* 2002; **33**:2631–2635.

Lees, K. R., Zivin, J. A., Ashwood, T. *et al.* Stroke-Acute Ischemic NXY Treatment (SAINT I) Trial Investigators. NXY-059 for acute ischemic stroke. *N. Engl. J. Med.* 2006; **354**:588–600.

Mayer, S. A. (2003) Ultra-early hemostatic therapy for intracerebral hemorrhage. *Stroke* 2003; **34**:224–229.

Poungvarin, N., Bhoopat, W., Viriyavejakul, A. *et al.* Effects of dexamethasone in primary supratentorial intracerebral hemorrhage. *N. Engl. J. Med.* 1987; **316**:1229–1233.

Smith, E. E. & Greenberg, S. M. Clinical diagnosis of cerebral amyloid angiopathy: validation of the Boston criteria. *Curr. Atheroscler. Rep.* 2003; **5**:260–266.

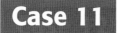

Worst headache of his life

Clinical history

A 54-year-old man had the sudden onset of the "worst headache" of his life and vomiting. The patient had arterial hypertension and was a moderate smoker: 30 pack–years (20 cig/day).

Examination

On admission, the patient was drowsy but had no focal neurological signs. Meningeal signs were negative. Blood pressure 170/900 mm Hg.

Neurological scores

NIH 0; Barthel Index 85; GCS: 15, Hunt and Hess: 1.

Special studies

Initial non-contrast CT showed hyperdense signal in the peripontine, basal, and posterior fossa cisterns as well as in the interhemispheric and Sylvian fissure. A conventional catheter angiography was performed, showing a saccular aneurysm of the ACA. The patient was operated on the same day and the aneurysm was clipped.

Follow-up

The patient was treated in the ICU and showed slightly elevated flow velocity measures of the intracerebral vessels between days 8 and 16. After 9 months, he was examined in the outpatient department and showed no focal neurological signs but symptoms of a minor depression.

Image findings

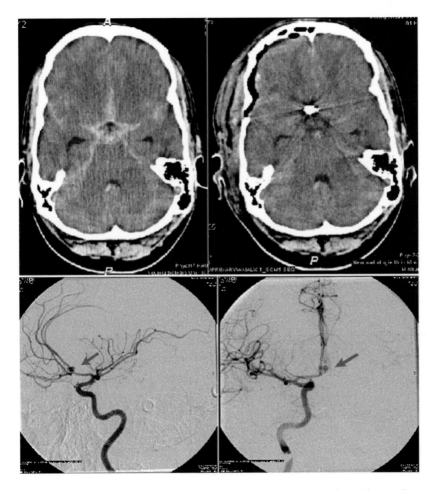

Figure 11.1 *Upper row left*: initial CT showing hyperdense signal of subarachnoid hemorrhage in the peripontine, basal and posterior fossa cisterns as well as the interhemispheric and Sylvian fissure. Bottom row: Conventional angiography showing saccular aneurysm of the ACA in different projections. *Upper row right*: Postsurgery CT showing the location of the clip.

Diagnosis

Subarachnoid hemorrhage due to ruptured aneurysm of the ACA.

General remarks

Intracranial aneurysms have been known to exist since ancient Egyptian times. The first report of a ruptured intracranial aneurysm as the cause of an

Table 11.1. *Hunt and Hess Classification*[a] *of Subarachnoid Hemorrhage*

Grade	Description	Peri-operative mortality (%)[b]	Probability of survival (%)[c]
0	Unruptured aneurysm		
1	Asymptomatic, or slight headache or nuchal rigidity	0–5	90
2	CN palsy, moderate or severe headache or nuchal rigidity	2–10	75
3	Slight focal deficit, lethargy, or confusion	10–15	65
4	Stupor, moderate or severe hemiparesis, early decerebrate posturing	60–70	45
5	Coma, decerebrate posturing, moribund	70–100	5

Notes:
[a] Modified from original paper. Add one grade for severe systemic disease or severe vasospasm.
[b] From Schubert (1993).
[c] From Archer *et al.* (1991).

subarachnoid hemorrhage was by John Blackhall of Oxford, England, in 1813. However, it was not until the end of the nineteenth century, due in part to the more detailed description of the signs and symptoms of subarachnoid hemorrhage and the technique of lumbar puncture developed by Quincke that the diagnosis of subarachnoid hemorrhage could be made prior to death.

Headache is the most common clinical symptom in subarachnoid hemorrhage, and occurs in 85% to 95% of patients. The headache is sudden and explosive in onset, often associated with nausea or vomiting, and is classically described as the "worst headache of one's life." Other symptoms include nuchal rigidity, seizures, photophobia, lethargy, and altered mentation. Brief loss of consciousness occurs in many patients at the time of hemorrhage, and is probably due to a sudden massive increase in intracranial pressure, with a resultant decrease or transient cessation of cerebral perfusion pressure. After subarachnoid hemorrhage, patients may recover fully or develop various levels of altered mentation. Persistent change in the level of consciousness may be due to intracerebral hemorrhage, hydrocephalus, persistently elevated intracranial pressure, or vasospasm.

Clinical signs that accompany the presenting symptoms often include a slight temperature elevation, hypertension, and ocular findings. Cranial nerve palsies and focal neurologic deficits may also be present, but are more often associated with aneurysmal subarachnoid hemorrhage (due to compression or embolic phenomenon, respectively). Finally, patients may present with various cardiac abnormalities, including chest pain, arrhythmias, ECG changes, and even full cardiopulmonary arrest. This presumably occurs due to a massive sympathetic discharge at the time of hemorrhage. The diagnosis of subarachnoid hemorrhage in such a situation should be reconsidered if the patient has no prior cardiac history and has persistent headaches, focal neurologic deficits, and papilledema.

Once a definitive diagnosis of subarachnoid hemorrhage has been made, patients are classified according to a standardized grading system. The Hunt and Hess classification is perhaps the best known and most widely used (Table 56.1). Analysis of data from the International Cooperative Aneurysm Study, however, failed to show any significant difference in outcomes between patients in grades 1 or 2 with normal level of conscience. Furthermore, they found that hemiparesis or aphasia had no effect on overall mortality rates. Therefore, the World Federation of Neurological Surgeons grading system has recently been recommended.

SUGGESTED READING

Archer, D. P., Shaw, D. A., Leblanc, R. L., & Tranmer, B. I. Haemodynamic considerations in the management of patients with subarachnoid haemorrhage. *Can. J. Anaesth.* 1991; **38**:454–470.

Diringer, M. N. To clip or to coil acutely ruptured intracranial aneurysms: update on the debate. *Curr. Opin. Crit. Care* 2005; **11**:121–125.

Edlow, J. A. & Caplan, L. R. Avoiding pitfalls in the diagnosis of subarachnoid hemorrhage. *N. Engl. J. Med.* 2000; **342**:29–36.

Fewel, M. E., Thompson, B. G. Jr., & Hoff, J. T. Spontaneous intracerebral hemorrhage: a review. *Neurosurg. Focus* 2003; **15**:E1.

Hunt, W. E. & Hess, R. M. Surgical risk as related to time of intervention in the repair of intracranial aneurysms. *J. Neurosurg.* 1968; **28**:14–20.

Naidech, A. M., Janjua, N., Kreiter, K. T. *et al.* Predictors and impact of aneurysm rebleeding after subarachnoid hemorrhage. *Arch. Neurol.* 2005; **62**:410–416.

Rosen, D. S. & Macdonald, R. L. Subarachnoid hemorrhage grading scales: a systematic review. *Neurocrit. Care* 2005; **2**:110–118.

Drooping eyelid and gait problems

Clinical history

A 47-year-old patient with no past neurological history reported gait imbalance and nausea since getting up in the morning that day. His wife noticed a drooping eyelid on the left. Apart from being a heavy smoker, there were no known risk factors or illnesses. He was not taking medication regularly.

Examination

Neurological examination showed slight left-sided limb ataxia, severe right-sided thermal and pain analgesia, and left Horner's syndrome with ptosis and miosis. Lingual and pharyngeal movements were normal. Muscle strength and discriminative sensibility were not affected. No cervical or occipital pain was present.

Neurological scores

NIH 4; Barthel Index 70; GCS 15.

Special studies

MRI showed a left dorsolateral medullary hyperintense lesion on diffusion- and T$_2$-weighted images. On MRA the left VA and PICA were not seen, while the contralateral VA and PICA were normal. Time-to-peak maps of the MR perfusion measurement showed hypoperfusion in the left PICA territory exceeding the area of the acute lesion. In the ultrasound examination of the cerebral vessels atherosclerosis was noted; the left V2 segment had a high resistance flow pattern indicating distal occlusion. No source of cardiac embolism or coagulation disorders were found. No MRI/ultrasound features or possible causes of a dissection were identified. The patient was treated with a platelet aggregation inhibitor.

Follow-up

On evaluation 4 months later the patient showed good recovery with slight imbalance and sensory deficits but overall independence in daily living.

Image Findings

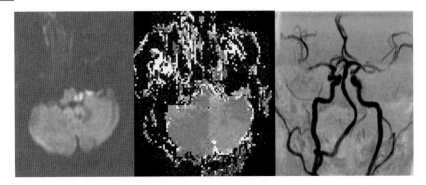

Figure 12.1 (a) DWI shows acute ischemia in the left dorsolateral medulla oblongata, while (b) PWI reveals a perfusion deficit of the left PICA territory. (c) Both ipsilateral VA and PICA are not seen on MRA (c).

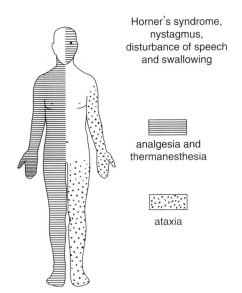

Horner's syndrome,
nystagmus,
disturbance of speech
and swallowing

analgesia and
thermanesthesia

ataxia

Figure 12.2 Clinical signs of Wallenberg's syndrome.

Diagnosis

Lateral medullary syndrome (Wallenberg's syndrome).

General remarks

Although not the first describer of the clinical features of lateral medullary infarction, Adolf Wallenberg became known for correlating clinical signs (1895) and postmortem localization of the lateral medullary lesion (1901). Although Wallenberg attributed the infarct to occlusion of PICA, his patient had an intracranial vertebral artery occlusion as well as PICA. Anatomical studies of Duvorney and others have shown that the lateral medulla is supplied almost exclusively by small penetrating arteries that originate from the intracranial vertebral arteries and course through the lateral medullary fossa to reach the lateral medulla. The medial branch of PICA supplies a small region in the dorsal medulla but not the lateral medulla. Of course, if the intracranial vertebral artery is abruptly occluded, the PICA territory will show decreased perfusion. Most lateral medullary infarcts are caused by intracranial vertebral artery occlusions. Only about one-fifth of lateral medullary infarcts are accompanied by PICA infarction.

Wallenberg's syndrome refers to a complex of symptoms caused by occlusion of the PICA or one of its branches supplying the lower and lateral portion of the brainstem. Typical signs at onset are severe vertigo, nausea, vomiting, ipsilateral ataxia, singultus, and dysphagia. Horner's syndrome is usually present. Deficits include sensory and sympathetic abnormalities, cerebellar, and pyramidal tract signs, and involvement of the cranial nerves V, IX, X, and XI. Vertebral artery dissection has been identified as an important cause of Wallenberg's syndrome, in some cases this has been linked to previous chiropractic manipulation.

Kim and coworkers found that heterogeneous MRI lesions in 37 patients with lateral medullary infarction were correlated with diverse angiographic findings, which in turn were thought to be due to different pathogenic mechanisms: etiology, location and size of the involved vessels, speed of the lesion development, and status of collaterals.

Even though thrombolysis in a case of lateral medullary syndrome has been reported recently, in most cases treatment for Wallenberg's syndrome is symptomatic. A feeding tube may be necessary if swallowing is very difficult. Speech/swallowing therapy may be beneficial. In some cases, medication may be used to reduce or eliminate pain. Some doctors report that the antiepileptic drug gabapentin appears to be an effective medication for individuals with chronic pain.

Special remarks

Unlike in acute stroke of the internal carotid artery territory, where vessel pathology can be demonstrated with ultrasound and MRA, the ability of both techniques might be limited to identifying obstructions of branches of the vertebral and basilar arteries. As shown in this case, the high contrast visualization with a combination of DWI and PWI can help to achieve the diagnosis of persistent vessel pathology and identify the extent of the abnormalities and tissue at risk for infarction in the posterior circulation.

FIRST DESCRIPTION

Anatomischer Befund in einem als "acute Bulbäraffection (Embolie der Arteria cerebelli posterior inferior sinistra.)" beschriebenen Falle. *Arch. Psychiatrie Nervenkrankh.*, Berlin, 1901; **34**:823.

Wallenberg, A. Akute Bulbäraffection (Embolie der Arteria cerebelli posterior inferior sinistra.). *Arch. Psychiatrie Nervenkrankh., Berlin*, 1895; **27**:504–540.

SUGGESTED READING

Caplan, L. R. *Posterior Circulation Disease: Clinical Features, Diagnosis, and Management,* Boston: Blackwell Science, 1996.

Caplan, L. R. Posterior circulation ischemia: then, now, and tomorrow. The Thomas Willis Lecture – 2000. *Stroke* 2000; **31**:2011–2023.

Duvernoy, H. M. *Human Brainstem Vessels.* Berlin: Springer-Verlag, 1978.

Fisher, C. M., Karnes, W. E., & Kubik, C. S. Lateral medullary infarction – the pattern of vascular occlusion. *J. Neuropath. Exp. Neurol.* 1961; **20**:323–379.

Hosoya, T., Watanabe, N., Yamaguchi, K., Kubota, H., & Onodera, Y. Intracranial vertebral artery dissection in Wallenberg syndrome. *Am. J. Neuroradiol.* 1994; **15**:1161–1165.

Khurana, D., Saini, M., Khandelwal, N., & Prabhakar, S. Thrombolysis in a case of lateral medullary syndrome: CT angiographic findings. *Neurology* 2005; **64**:1232.

Kim, J. S., Lee, J. H., & Choi, C. G. Patterns of lateral medullary infarction: vascular lesion-magnetic resonance imaging correlation of 34 cases. *Stroke* 1998; **29**:645–652.

Pearce, J. M. Wallenberg's syndrome. *J. Neurol. Neurosurg. Psychiatry* 2000; **68**:570.

Sacco, R. L., Freddo, L., Bello, J. A., Odel, J. G., Onesti, S. T., & Mohr, J. P. Wallenberg's lateral medullary syndrome. Clinical-magnetic resonance imaging correlations. *Arch. Neurol.* 1993; **50**:609–614.

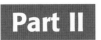

Part II

Uncommon cases of stroke

Similar infarction – different outcome: the importance of the brain network

Clinical history

Case a

A 38-year-old dentist described a transient attack characterized by vertigo, nausea, and blurred vision lasting for 2 minutes while playing golf. Despite the very short episode, he came to the emergency room, where neurological examination on admission showed normal gait. The only abnormality was a slight veering to the left when he walked and slight hypotonia of the left arm when he was asked to quickly lower his arm, stopping it abruptly.

He had no past important medical illnesses or risk factors.

Neurological scores

NIH 0; Barthel Index 100; GCS 15.

Case b

A 78-year-old man came to the emergency room 5 hours after the acute onset of severe gait ataxia, vertigo, and nausea. He had no previous history of neurological symptoms and had been completely independent. The clinical examination showed dysarthria, and nystagmus to the right side. Heel–shin and finger–nose testing were dysmetric on the left. The patient was not able to stand or walk by himself. He reported arterial hypertension, hyperlipidemia, coronary heart disease since 6 years ago, myocardial infarct 2 years ago.

Neurological scores

NIH 6; Barthel Index 30; GCS 15.

Special studies

Case a

Because of the clear description of his symptoms and their localization to the brainstem/cerebellum, MRI was performed immediately. Diffusion-weighted imaging showed an acute infarct in the territory of the lateral branch of the left

PICA with no pre-existent infra- or supratentorial lesions. Extensive evaluation including ECD, TCD, MRA, functional transcranial ultrasound, thoracic and transesophageal echocardiography, Holter-ECG and blood testing were normal.

Case b

Diffusion-weighted imaging showed an acute infarct in the left inferior cerebellar artery territory involving the vermis in the distribution of the medial branch of PICA and additional severe white matter changes with periventricular rims and caps. Severe macroangiopathy with occlusion of the left vertebral artery and high grade stenosis of the right vertebral artery, occlusion of the left ICA and a 70% stenosis of the right ICA was found in addition.

Follow-up

Case a

The patient left hospital without neurological deficits and able to walk normally. He had no further strokes. Secondary prophylactic therapy consisted of aspirin.

Case b

After 23 days, the patient was sent to a rehabilitation center because of persistent gait ataxia and vertigo. The patient was treated at this time with aspirin.

Diagnosis

Acute PICA infarctions: outcome is influenced by supratentorial white matter lesions.

General remarks

The cerebellar vermis and adjacent nodulus and flocculus contain important connections with the vestibular nuclei in the brainstem. When the vermis is infracted in the territory of the medial branch of PICA the symptoms and signs include severe vertigo and gait ataxia mimicking a vestibular syndrome. Gait ataxia may be severe but if unassociated with other brain lesions it usually improves during 3 to 6 months. Lateral cerebellar lesions in the distribution of the lateral branch of PICA cause mostly slight limb hypotonia and have only a minor influence on gait. Vertigo is usually not severe and transient.

Image findings

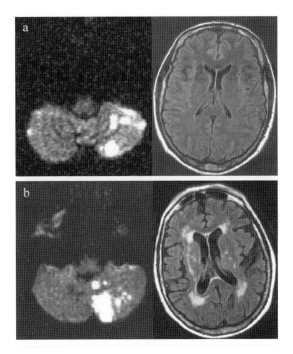

Figure 13.1 Acute PICA infarction (DWI): patient 1 (a) infarction of the lateral inferior cerebellum sparing the vermis with no supratentorial white matter disease, patient 2 (b) infarction of the inferior cerebellar vermis with severe supratentorial white matter disease.

Branch territory cerebellar infarcts are usually due to embolism either from the heart or aorta or from the vertebral arteries. In the second patient the embolus likely arose from his severe vertebral artery disease in the neck. In the first patient a plaque or minor vertebral artery dissection not imagable with current techniques was likely responsible.

Special remarks

Stroke signs and symptoms have traditionally been analysed with regard to lesion localization, infarct size and underlying stroke mechanism. However, the detection of subcortical white matter lesions (WML) on MRI has only rarely been taken into consideration. Both increasing age and vascular risk factors like hypertension, diabetes and hyperhomocysteinemia are related to the degree of

WML. The clinical relevance of WML is controversial, however, recent data confirm the coexistence of vascular dementia, gait unsteadiness and urinary incontinence subsumed in the syndrome of SVE with severe white matter lesions. The fact that isolated cerebellar infarctions in general have a good functional outcome compared to infarctions in other vascular territories is well established. We have found that bad clinical outcome in patients with isolated cerebellar stroke strongly correlates with the presence of supratentorial WML as seen in these two patients.

While almost identical acute lesions occurred in both patients without history of neurological deficits, patient 1 experienced only transient symptoms, while patient 2 suffered from persistent clinical deficits. The difference between the two patients has therefore to be sought at the level of compensatory mechanisms and the disruption of pre-existing networks. The non-focal character suggests an important function of subcortical relay stations and connecting fibers to compensate for cerebellar lesions evidenced by loss of network compensation in white matter disease. Thus the most prominent feature of age seems to be the loss of network function as indicated by the detection of WML.

SUGGESTED READING

Baezner, H. & Hennerici, M. From trepidant abasia to motor network failure–gait disorders as a consequence of subcortical vascular encephalopathy (SVE): review of historical and contemporary concepts. *J. Neurol. Sci.* 2005; 229–230:81–8.

Caplan, L. R. Cerebellar infarcts. In *Posterior Circulation Vascular Disease: Clinical Features, Diagnosis, and Management.* Boston: Blackwell Science, 1996.

Chaves, C. J., Caplan, L. R., Chung, C.-S., & Amarenco, P. Cerebellar infarcts. In Appel, S. (ed). *Current Neurology,* Vol. 14, St Louis: Mosby-Year Book, 1994; 143–177.

Chaves, C. J., Caplan, L. R., Chung, C.-S. *et al.* Cerebellar infarcts in the New England Medical Center Posterior Circulation Stroke Registry. *Neurology* 1994; **44**:1385–1390.

Grips, E., Sedlaczek, O., Bazner, H., Fritzinger, M., Daffertshofer, M., & Hennerici, M. Supratentorial age-related white matter changes predict outcome in cerebellar stroke. *Stroke* 2005; **36**:1988–1993.

Kase, C. S., Norrving, B., Levine, S. R. *et al.* Cerebellar infarction. Clinical and anatomic observations in 66 cases. *Stroke* 1993; **24**:76–83.

Kelly, P. J., Stein, J., Shafqat, S. *et al.* Functional recovery after rehabilitation for cerebellar *Stroke.* 2001; **32**:530–534.

Taylor, W. D., MacFall, J. R., Provenzale, J. M. *et al.* Serial MR imaging of volumes of hyperintense white matter lesions in elderly patients: correlation with vascular risk factors. *Am. J. Roentgenol.* 2003; **181**:571–576.

An 80-year-old woman with sudden paresis and normal motor latencies

Clinical history

An 80-year-old woman was brought to the emergency room by paramedics because of a sudden weakness of the right limbs and a loss of ability to speak. Assuming an acute stroke in the left middle cerebral artery territory, the patient was admitted to the Stroke Unit.

General history

Ablation of the right breast due to cancer 5 years earlier, no known cerebrovascular risk factors.

Examination

On neurological examination, the patient was slightly drowsy but arousable, had intact language comprehension but no language production or articulation. Reading or writing could not be tested. There was a severe sensorimotor hemiparesis on the right side.

Neurological scores

NIH 12; Barthel Index 40; GCS 13.

Special studies

MRI showed an acute ischemic lesion in the left ACA territory and occlusion of the left A2 segment. Despite thorough examinations, no potential source of embolism was found. There were no signs of metastases or paraneoplastic illness (incl. negative antibodies Anti-Hu, Ri, Yo). Somewhat surprisingly, motor-evoked potentials showed normal bilateral motor conduction time.

Follow-up

One week after the event, the patient was awake, fully oriented, had normal comprehension, and no aphasia or dysarthria. She spoke very slowly and quietly, almost whispering. There was residual hemiparesis on the right with only slight signs of motor neglect.

Image findings

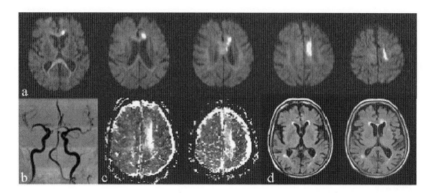

Figure 14.1 (a) Diffusion-weighted images show acute left ACA stroke in the territory of the pericallosal artery. (b) MRA shows occlusion of the left ACA in the A2 segment. (c) Perfusion MRI with hypoperfusion in the left ACA territory, also affecting not infarcted midline regions. (d) T_2-weighted FLAIR images show slight periventricular chronic lesions.

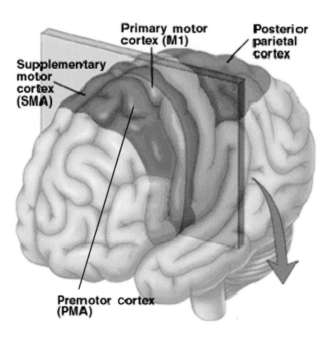

Figure 14.2 Principal cortical domains of the motor system. (Adapted from www.brainconnection.com)

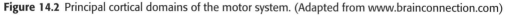

Diagnosis

Mutism, hemiparesis, and hemineglect in a patient with anterior cerebral artery stroke.

General remarks

The territory of the ACA was first studied by Heubner* and Duret in 1874. Foix and Hillemand reported the first clinical syndromes of ACA stroke based on clinico-pathologic studies in the 1920s. In 1990 the first large clinical-CT study from the Lausanne Stroke Registry was published showing that the etiologic spectrum of ACA stroke was very similar to that of middle cerebral artery infarcts. In a recent MRI study of 48 patients with acute ACA stroke, the authors reported three main clinical patterns depending on lesion side:

(a) left-side infarction consisting of mutism, transcortical motor aphasia, and hemiparesis with lower limb predominance;
(b) right-side infarction accompanied by acute confusional state, motor hemi-neglect and hemiparesis; and
(c) bilateral infarction presenting with akinetic mutism, severe sphincter dysfunction, and dependent functional outcome.

Special remarks

The pericallosal artery originates from the A2 segment of the ACA and follows the superior surface of the corpus callosum. It supplies the medial and superior surfaces of the posterior part of the parietal lobe and can affect parts of the supplementary motor area. The supplementary motor area is located above and medial to the premotor cortex, and is considered to play an important role in planning, initiating and maintaining sequential motor actions. Lesions involving the left supplementary motor area have been described to cause acute confusional states, mutism, abulia and even transcortical motor aphasia. Disturbances of the supplementary motor area, however, have only rarely been reported to cause severe and always transient contralateral hemiplegia. Commonly, in ACA stroke motor symptoms predominating the lower limb occur in lesions of the precentral region, while more facio-brachial predominance is a result of occlusion of the recurrent artery of Heubner involving the internal capsule. The fact that, in our

---

* Heubner's artery (synonym: Recurrent artery of Heubner, medial striate artery) supplies the anteromedial part of the head of the caudate and anteroinferior internal capsule. It is the largest of the medial lenticulostriate arteries which typically arises from the proximal A2 or A1 segment. Named after Johann Otto Leonhard Heubner, German pediatrician (1843–1926).

patient, hemiparesis was not a result of pyramidal weakness was readily confirmed by MEP examination, and it could only in part be explained by neglect. We assume that the lesion in the supplementary motor area resulted in severe disturbance of motor function possibly aggravated by involvement of parts of the adjacent premotor cortex (Freund, 1987).

FIRST DESCRIPTION

Duret, H. Recherches anatomiques sur la circulation de l'encéphale. *Arch. Physiol. Norm. Path.* 1874; **2**:919–957.

Foix, C. & Hillemand, P. Les syndromes de l'artère antérieure. *Encéphale* 1925; **20**:209–232.

Heubner, O. *Die luetische Erkrankung der Hirnarterien.* Leipzig: FCW Vogel, 1874.

CURRENT REVIEW

Kumral, E., Bayulkem, G., Evyapan, D., & Yunten, N. Spectrum of anterior cerebral artery territory infarction: clinical and MRI findings. *Eur. J. Neurol.* 2002; **9**:615–624.

SUGGESTED READING

Bogousslavsky, J. & Regli, F. Anterior cerebral artery territory infarction in the Lausanne Stroke Registry. Clinical and etiologic patterns. *Arch. Neurol.* 1990; **47**:144–150.

Freund, H.-J. Abnormalities of motor behavior after cortical lesions in humans. In *Handbook of Physiology,* Section 1 The Nervous System, Vol. 5 Part 2, American Physiological Society, Bethesda 1987; 763–810.

Geschwind, N. & Kaplan, E. (1962). A human deconnection syndrome: a preliminary report. *Neurology* 1962; **12**:675–685.

Lower limb weakness after surgery

Clinical history

A 43-year-old male was treated for infiltrating carcinoma of the bladder by radical resection of the bladder, prostate, and seminal vesicles with *en bloc* lymphadenectomy followed by formation of an ileal bladder. To maintain postoperative analgesia, an epidural catheter (20-G) was introduced between the 3rd and 4th lumbar laminae, and tested in its epidural site with an injection of 5 ml 0.5% bupivacaine preoperatively. The operation lasted 10 h. Throughout the operation, the patient was placed in a hyperlordotic supine position with a 17 degrees head- and trunk-down tilt (vertex at L1) and the legs extended 17 degrees at the hips to raise the pubis. Continuous intraarterial monitoring of systemic blood pressure documented 90/50 mmHg as the lowest recording. Throughout the procedure, the systolic pressure was less than 100 mmHg for only 15 min during the premedication phase. Blood loss of 7 liters during the operation was replaced by autologous blood, fresh frozen plasma, 0.9% NaCl, and colloids. Toward the end of the operation, 10 mg morphine in 10 ml 0.9% NaCl was instilled through the epidural catheter, and 2 h later, 0.25% bupivacaine was started at a rate of 4 ml/h, after an initial test dose of 4 ml 0.5% bupivacaine. The patient was sedated, and his lungs were ventilated until the following morning, when after awakening, he complained of complete loss of sensation in the left lower limb and right leg and foot.

Examination

Neurologic examination showed severe weakness of both lower limbs. The patient was unable to stand.

Special studies

Initially, this was thought to be due to the pharmacologic action of bupivacaine, but the weakness persisted when the epidural analgesia was discontinued on the third postoperative day. A plain T1w and T2w MRI scan of the lumbar spine on the 3rd day and a plain and gadolinium T1w MRI scan of the lumbar and thoracic spine on the fourth day showed no spinal cord abnormality. However, in the dorsal third of the vertebral bodies of L2 and L3, an area of hyperintense signal was visible in T2w and T1w images (a), (b). The same day, examination of cerebrospinal fluid showed lymphocytosis (22/µl), a slightly elevated total protein (0.97 g/l, Lowry) and no intrathecal IgG production, indicating a partial break-down of blood–cerebrospinal fluid barrier.

Image findings

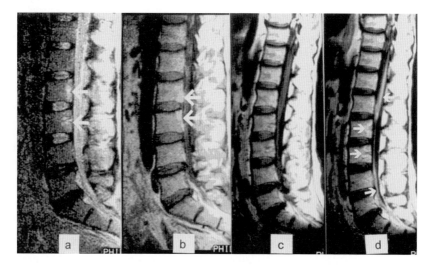

Figure 15.1 MRI scans of the lumbar spine on the 3rd day: (a) T_2-weighted and (b) T_1-weighted. Hyperintense signal in the dorsal third of the vertebral bodies of L2 and L3, consistent with infarction. On the 27th day T1-weighted sagittal MRI without (c) and with (d) gadolinium shows enhancement of lumbosacral spinal cord and dura mater and less enhancement of the vertebral bodies L2 and L3.

Diagnosis

Lumbar spinal cord infarction due to operation in the hyperlordotic position.

Special remarks

In this patient, a lesion of the cauda equina or the spinal cord was likely because paraplegia occurred with impairment of perianal sensation and incontinence.

However, due to the arterial supply of the lumbosacral spinal cord, the typical anterior spinal artery syndrome with dissociated sensory loss of pinprick and temperature sensation was – as usual – not present. Electrophysiologic testing proved an anterior horn or root lesion and, concerning the sensory pathways, a supraganglionic site of the lesion. It was 4 weeks after onset and 2 weeks after clearly diagnostic electrophysiologic results that contrast-enhanced T1w MRI showed the infarction of the spinal cord; at this time DWI MRI was unavailable. However, in the initial MRI, the abnormal signal of the dorsal aspects of the vertebral bodies of L2 and L3 1(c) could have been interpreted as ischemic bone infarction. The slight CSF pleocytosis could be explained by the large extent of the ischemia.

Because the dura mater and the posterior vertebral bodies are supplied by branches of more than one radicular artery along their intraspinal courses, an increase of intraspinal pressure resulting in a sealing-off effect of the foramina intervertebralia must be considered etiologically. The vertebral infarctions located in the dorsal aspects of the vertebral bodies support this suggestion. The assumed increased intraspinal pressure could have resulted from inferior vena cava (IVC) compression because of the hyperlordotic supine position, as previously suggested for other cases in the literature. However, IVC or iliac vein compression due to surgical packs or retractors cannot be excluded. Local anesthetic was not given during the operation but in small quantities thereafter. Accidental injection of local anesthetic into the subarachnoid space was unlikely because the blood pressure had remained stable. More likely, epidural analgesia played no causative role in the development of spinal cord infarction in this case.

General remarks

The occurrence of paraplegia after various surgical procedures performed during perioperative epidural analgesia or anesthesia was estimated to be 1:11 000. In many cases, immediate postoperative paraparesis was attributed to a direct toxic effect of the local anesthetic or acute ischemia. A neurotoxic effect can be postulated if the highly concentrated anesthetic used for epidural analgesia has been injected inadvertently into the subarachnoid space. Ischemic lesions of intraspinal nervous tissue can be caused by a decrease in systemic BP, direct damage to radicular spinal arteries, or an increase in intraspinal pressure. The latter situation can occur after injection of large amounts of local anesthetic via an epidural catheter or IVC compression, e.g., due to surgical packs and retractors, a pregnant womb, or a patient's hyperlordotic position. Under these circumstances, the presence of a lumbar spinal canal stenosis can facilitate the increase of intraspinal pressure. The diagnosis of spinal cord ischemia is now greatly enhanced by available DWI and ADC MRI, so that it can often be visualized within the first 48 hours. In the absence of clear changes of the spinal cord the demonstration of infarction of the vertebral spine or intervertebral discs can sometimes aid the diagnosis.

FIRST DESCRIPTION

Urquhart-Hay, D. Paraplegia following epidural analgesia. *Anaesthesia* 1969; **24**:461–470.

CURRENT REVIEW

Roberts, D. R. D., Roe, J., & Baudouin, C. Hyperlordosis as a possible factor in the development of spinal cord infarction. *Br. J. Anaesth.* 2003; **90**:797–800.

SUGGESTED READING

Amoiridis, G., Ameridou, I., & Mavridis, M. Intervertebral disk and vertebral body infarction as a confirmatory sign of spinal cord ischemia. *Neurology* 2004; **63**:1755.

Bromage, P. R. "Paraplegia following epidural analgesia": a misnomer. *Anaesthesia* 1976; **31**:947–949.

Gass, A., Back, T., Behrens, S., & Maras, A. MRI in spinal cord infarction. *Neurology* 2000; **54**:2195.

Küker, W., Weller, M., Klose, U., Krapf, H., Dichgans, J., & Nägele, T. Diffusion-weighted MRI of spinal cord infarction – high resolution imaging and time course of diffusion abnormality. *J. Neurol.* 2004; **251**:818–824.

Teague, C. A. & Urquhart-Hay, D. Spinal thrombophlebitis after prostatectomy with hypotensive anaesthesia: a case report. *NZ Med. J.* 1974; **80**:654.

Usubiaga, J. E. Neurological complications following epidural anesthesia. *Int. Anesthesiol. Clin.* 1975; **13**:1–153.

Yuh, W. T. C., Marsh, E. E., Wang, A. K. *et al.* MR imaging of spinal cord and vertebral body infarction. *Am. J. Neuroradiol.* 1992; **13**:145–154.

A young engineer with suspected MS

Clinical history

A previously healthy 45-year-old engineer with a 1 week history of headache, malaise, and flu-like symptoms presented with progressive unexplained apathy and sub-acute cognitive decline, disabling him from proceeding with his professional and daily life activities.

Examination

On examination, he gave an accurate history, but appeared slow mentally and on motor examination, while the neurologic examination was otherwise normal on formal testing.

Special studies

Laboratory evaluation showed possible indications of slight inflammation (WBC 11.7×10 E^-9, C-reactive protein 12 mg/l) and a lumbar puncture was performed to investigate possible inflammatory disease in the CSF, showing slightly elevated cell count (5) and protein (637 mg/l). The initial CT scan showed multiple hypodense areas bilaterally in the periventricular and deep subcortical white matter and inflammatory-demyelinating disease (e.g., MS, ADEM) was thought to be the most likely diagnosis at this point. However, MRI and Doppler ultrasound findings changed this view substantially. While T_2-weighted MRI confirmed bilateral subcortical T_2-hyperintense white matter lesions (inkeeping with inflammatory-demyelinating disease), DWI and PWI identified those areas as acute ischemic lesions, located exactly in hemodynamic risk zones of both MCA territories. MRA revealed bilateral lack of flow signal in the ICA and reduction of flow signal in both MCAs, corresponding well to signs of marked hypoperfusion on PWI. T_1-weighted MRI after contrast showed no enhancement. Further T_2-weighted sequences showed vessel wall hematoma of both ICAs, while Doppler/Duplex-ultrasound examination confirmed bilateral ICA dissections with evidence of bidirectional high resistance flow.

Follow-up

On 6-month follow-up, there was complete clinical recovery.

Image findings

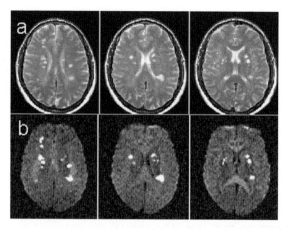

Figure 16.1 T$_2$-weighted and DWI axial images at presentation. Bilateral subcortical hyperintense lesions are noted on T$_2$-weighted (a) slices and DWI (b) shows corresponding hyperintense signal change and reduced apparent diffusion coefficients (*not shown*).

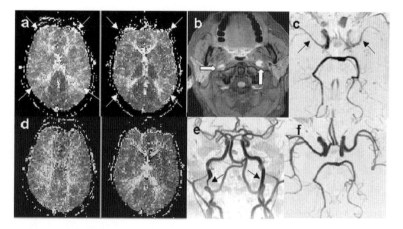

Figure 16.2 PWI and MRA at presentation and on follow-up. On time-to-peak-maps (a) delay of contrast-bolus-arrival is indicated by bright signal both in middle cerebral artery and anterior cerebral artery territories (arrows), while posterior cerebral artery territory, including occipital parenchyma and the thalami, clearly show earlier contrast bolus arrival as indicated by darker signal. This is normalized on follow-up time- to-peak maps. (b) A T$_1$-weighted-fat-suppressed image demonstrates hyperintensity within the lumen of the ICA

Diagnosis

Bilateral internal carotid artery dissection with bilateral subcortical acute ischemic lesions.

General remarks

It is now widely acknowledged that spontaneous dissections of the extracranial vessels are an important source of cerebral ischemia. While the overall frequency is 2.6 to 2.9 per 100 000, dissection of the internal carotid artery accounts for up to 20% of ischemic events in younger patients with a peak in the fifth decade, often in the absence of vascular risk factors.

Special remarks

Dissection of the internal carotid artery may be difficult to diagnose on the basis of historical information and clinical signs only and even standard brain imaging (CT, T_2-weighted MRI) may not be sufficient to delineate the underlying pathology clearly as shown in this case. The clinical symptoms and parenchymal lesion pattern on CT were suggestive of inflammatory-demyelinating disease, but MRA, DWI and PWI revealed acute ischemic lesions, bilateral internal carotid artery obstruction, and bilateral hypoperfusion in the MCA territories, which was confirmed by Doppler/Duplex ultrasound.

SUGGESTED READING

Baumgartner, R. W., Arnold, M., Baumgartner, I. *et al.* Carotid dissection with and without ischemic events: local symptoms and cerebral artery findings. *Neurology* 2001; **57**:827–832.

Biousse, V., D'Anglejan-Chatillon, J., Touboul, P. J. *et al.* Time course of symptoms in extracranial carotid artery dissections. A series of 80 patients. *Stroke* 1995; **26**:235–239.

Gass, A., Szabo, K., Lanczik, O., & Hennerici, M. G. Magnetic resonance imaging assessment of carotid artery dissection. *Cerebrovasc. Dis.* 2002; **13**:70–73.

Schevink, W. I. Spontaneous dissection of the carotid and vertebral arteries. *N. Engl. J. Med.* 2001; **344**:898–906.

Caption for Fig. 16.2 (*cont.*)
indicating vessel wall hematoma with a minimal residual flow-void phenomenon (dark dot). This is confirmed on MRA (c) that shows faint flow signal in both MCA and ICA in the axial projection 3D image. On follow-up, MRA shows restoration of flow in both ICAs and MCAs at the level of the circle of Willis (f) while on coronal views (e) there is still some residual narrowing of the ICA at the level of the base of the skull (arrows).

Vertigo after lifting a heavy suitcase

Clinical history

A 45-year-old man noticed acute severe pain in the right shoulder after lifting a heavy suitcase. Shortly after, he developed 15 seconds of non-motion directed vertigo. Later, travelling by train in a sitting position – except for minor persisting pain in the shoulder – he felt well. After a symptom-free interval of 4 hours, all of a sudden he reported a transient loss of spatial orientation and a feeling like being shaken in an aeroplane during severe turbulence. Apparently he had involuntarily moved in his seat, thus catching bedazzled looks from fellow train passengers. During this episode he had no diplopia, nausea, or visual disturbances. After a few minutes, he recovered completely apart from persisting pain in the right shoulder and neck.

General history was unrevealing.

Examination

Orthopedic consultation and neurologic examination 5 hours after onset of symptoms was normal, at this time the pain was subsiding.

Neurological scores

NIH 0; Barthel 100; GCS 15.

Special studies

Electronystagmography showed a minimally decreased downward optokinetic nystagmus. Extracranial Doppler/Duplex sonography and MR-angiography confirmed a dissection of the right vertebral artery as suspected from the acute pain syndrome. DW-MRI, ADC and FLAIR studies revealed an unexpected unique small acute infarction of 2 mm diameter in the center of the cerebellar vermis. By means of perfusion imaging techniques, the vascular territory affected by the dissection could be identified: time-to-peak maps showed a late arrival of the contrast media in the complete right PICA-territory.

Image findings

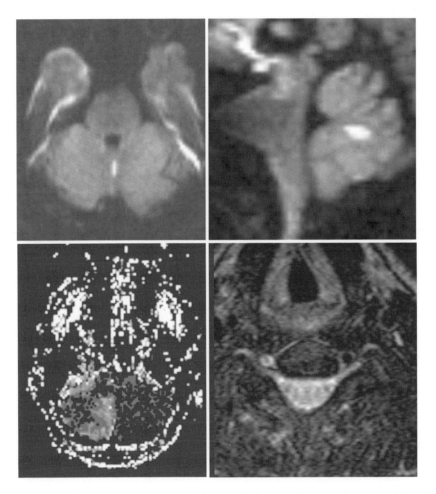

Figure 17.1 Top row: infarction in the center of the cerebellar vermis on DWI in the axial (*left*) and sagittal plane (*right*). *Bottom row*: perfusion-weighted imaging (*left*) indicates delayed contrast agent bolus arrival in the right PICA territory due to a dissection of the right vertebral artery seen on fat-saturated axial T$_2$-weighted images showing arterial wall hematoma (*right*).

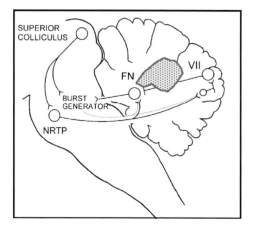

Figure 17.2 Schematic drawing of the MR-DWI lesion in the center of the cerebellar vermis (sagittal projection) vs. the fastigial nucleus and the critical cerebellar projection area (VII). Further components: nucleus reticularis tegmenti pontis, saccadic burst generator.

Diagnosis

Vertebral artery dissection with infarction in the center of the cerebellar vermis.

General remarks

Heterogeneous sources and etiologies cause vertigo and diagnosis is often difficult in the absence of characteristic signs in patients with transient symptoms. A history of sudden onset vertigo associated with a loss of spatial orientation – though very transient and non-directed – is indicative of acute cerebellar stroke. By the time of clinical presentation, cerebellar signs may already have improved. Although the lesion site may vary, the syndrome is certainly underestimated due to often scant history taking in emergency room settings and insufficient imaging protocols.

Special remarks

Spatial disorientation and severe vertigo without motion-related patterns are characteristic for an involvement of the cerebellar vermis and may be identified by meticulous clinical history taking and imaging studies. In this patient the tiny lesion in the midline was accidentally mistaken to be an MR – artefact. Only after insisting on the relevance of clinical symptoms could a second scan confirm the lesion. The fastigial nuclei close to the medullary center of the vermis integrate afferences from the vermiform cortices, the vestibular nuclei, and the accessory olives and have efferences via the lower cerebellar peduncles back to the vestibular nuclei. They are the major cerebellar relay centers mediating cerebellar inhibition on the vestibular system. The acute ischemic lesion observed in this patient fits both the fastigial nucleus and its afferent tracts from the vermiform cortex (VII).

CURRENT REVIEW

Tatu, L., Moulin, T., Bogousslavsky, J., & Duvernoy, H. Arterial territories of human brain: brainstem and cerebellum. *Neurology* 1996; **47**:1125–1135.

SUGGESTED READING

Scudder, C. A. Role of the fastigial nucleus in controlling horizontal saccades during adaptation. *Ann. NY Acad. Sci.* 2002; **978**:63–78.

Wearne, S., Raphan, T., & Cohen, B. Control of spatial orientation of the angular vestibuloocular reflex by the nodulus and uvula. *J. Neurophysiol.* 1998; **79**:2690–2715.

A 79-year-old man with a typical MCA-stroke?

Clinical history

A 79-year-old man was admitted to the Stroke Unit because of slurred speech and left-side limb weakness that he had noticed upon awakening in the morning. Extensive outpatient examinations had been performed 4 months earlier due to dizziness and exertional dyspnea with normal findings in ECG, stress ECG, transthoracic echocardiography, carotid ultrasound and cranial CT.

Medical history revealed mild but untreated arterial hypertension over the previous 10 years.

Examination

On neurological examination, the patient had dysarthria, a left facial weakness and a left sensorimotor hemiparesis.

Special studies

CT showed a typical small anterior division right MCA territory infarction of embolic origin, likely due to previously undiagnosed non-valvular atrial fibrillation. ECG-monitoring detected intermittent atrial fibrillation. Duplex ultrasound of the carotid arteries revealed only slight signs of arteriosclerosis. Transesophageal echocardiography, however, showed a right atrial tumor, suggestive for either thrombus or myxoma. A few microbubbles appeared in the left atrium, although only after more than three heart cycles. Thoracic CT proved a right atrial tumor invading the right atrial myocardium and extending into the superior vena cava as well as pericardial and right-sided pleural effusions. After surgical removal of the tumor, the histological examination surprisingly revealed a primary cardiac Non-Hodgkin's lymphoma. The immunohistochemical classification showed a diffuse large B-cell lymphoma with high IgM expression.

Follow-up

An extensive diagnostic evaluation yielded no evidence of an extracardiac lymphoma manifestation. The patient refused all therapy and died 6 weeks later at home.

Image findings

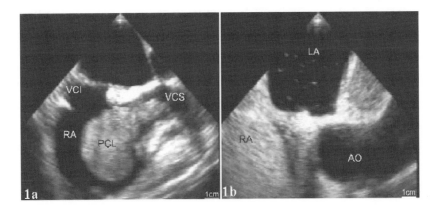

Figure 18.1 (a) Transesophageal echocardiography shows a primary cardiac lymphoma (PCL) in the right atrium extending into the superior vena cava (VCS). RA indicates right atrium, VCI inferior vena cava. (b) Contrast transesophageal echocardiography yields moderate right-to-left shunting of microbubbles only in a late phase after opacification of the right atrium. LA indicates left atrium, AO aorta.

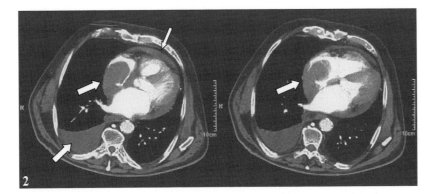

Figure 18.2 Thoracic CT shows primary cardiac lymphoma in the right atrium invading the myocardium (white arrows) as well as pericardial (thin gray arrow) and pleural effusions (thick gray arrow).

Diagnosis

Embolic stroke caused by right atrial primary cardiac lymphoma.

General remarks

The most common primary cardiac tumor is the atrial myxoma, which accounts for 40%–50% of all these neoplasms. The other tumors of the pathological spectrum include benign and malignant cell types. The overall incidence of the disease is low, and found in 0.0001%–0.5% in autopsy series. Benign tumors include myxomas, rhabdomyoma, fibroma, fibroelastoma, hemangioma, lipoma, teratoma, and hamartoma. Malignant tumors are generally sarcomatous in nature. Primary cardiac lymphoma is defined as the only manifestion of a malignant lymphoma. This condition is extremely rare; there are only about 100 cases described in literature. Treated with the standard chemotherapy (CHOP: cyclophosphamide, doxorubicin, vincristine, and prednisone) prognosis is unfavorable, with a mortality of 60% within 6 months.

Special remarks

In this patient, primary cardiac lymphoma presents the unique origin of stroke. Two different pathophysiological mechanisms are conceivable: The dilatation of the right atrium may have caused atrial fibrillation predisposing to cardioembolism. Alternatively, although rather unlikely, increased thrombogenicity due to turbulent flow and the large surface of the tumor in the right atrium may have facilitated a paradoxical embolism either through a small PFO or a pulmonary shunt.

CURRENT REVIEW

Ikeda, H., Nakamura, S., Nishimaki, H. *et al.* Primary lymphoma of the heart. Case report and literature review, *Path. Int.* 2004; **54**:187–195.

SUGGESTED READING

Gowda, R. M. & Khan, I. A., Clinical perspectives of primary cardiac lymphoma, *Angiology* 2003; **54**:599–604.

Quigley, M. M., Schwartzman, E., Boswell, P. D. *et al.* A unique atrial primary cardiac lymphoma mimicking myxoma presenting with embolic stroke: a case report, *Blood* 2003; **101**:4708–4710.

Rolla, G., Bertero, M. T., Pastena, G. *et al.* Primary lymphoma of the heart. A case report and review of the literature, *Leuk. Res.* 2002; **26**:117–120.

Ryu, S. J., Choi, B. W., & Choe, K. O. CT and MR findings of primary cardiac lymphoma: report upon 2 cases and review, *Yonsei Med. J.* 2001; **42**:451–456.

A man with slowly progressive weakness of the left hand

Clinical history

A 67-year-old man described slowly progressive weakness of the left hand during a period of 10 days. Symptoms had started with slight weakness of the hand when grasping an object and had increased to sudden dropping and finally complete palsy of the left hand.

General history

Hypertension since 2 years before, diabetes, hypercholesterolemia.

Examination

Clinical examination showed a left-sided sensorimotor hemiparesis, with brachiofacial and distal accentuation of weakness, and dysarthria.

Neurological scores

NIH 8; Barthel Index 60; GCS 15.

Special studies

Cranial MRI showed multiple T_2-hyperintense lesions in the anterior, internal and posterior border zone regions of the MCA territory, identified by DWI as acute ischemic lesions with emphasis in the subcortical region. PWI showed moderate hypoperfusion in the complete territory of the right MCA, accentuated in the acute ischemic areas. On MRA a severe proximal stenosis of the right MCA was found, confirmed by subsequent Doppler/Duplex-ultrasound examination with a proximal stenosis of the right MCA (maximal velocity 3 m/s). Furthermore, generalized arteriosclerotic changes causing a moderately severe stenosis of the left ICA and the basilar artery were found. Transthoracic echocardiography and functional transcranial ultrasound excluded cardiac and other vascular sources of embolism.

Follow-up

The patient was treated with an antiplatelet agent (clopidogrel) for secondary prophylaxis. About 20 months following the initial stroke, the patient was readmitted to the hospital with a worsening of the residual left-sided sensorimotor hemiparesis and mild dysarthria. MRI-scan showed in turn multiple acute ischemic lesions in both the subcortical and cortical regions of the right MCA territory and the previously diagnosed MCA pathology.

Image findings

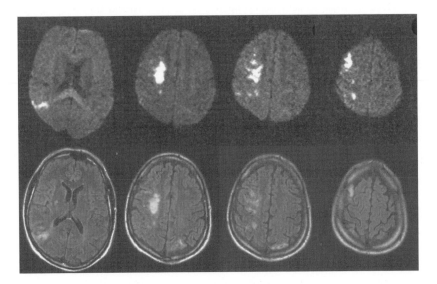

Figure 19.1 Diffusion-weighted imaging (DWI, *upper row*) performed on day 4 after initial stroke shows multiple chainlike acute ischemic lesions along the anterior and posterior border zone regions and additional small acute cortical lesions in the territory of the right MCA. T$_2$-weighted FLAIR technique shows additional chronic lesion in the left posterior MCA region.

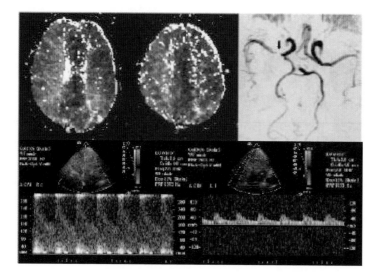

Figure 19.2 PWI (*upper row left and middle*) with time-to-peak maps show slight delay of contrast agent bolus arrival in the complete territory of the right MCA, most pronounced in the acute ischemic areas. In addition hypoperfusion in the posterior border zone region of the left MCA was caused by the moderate stenosis of the left distal ICA. MRA (*upper row, right*) shows proximal stenosis of the right MCA (arrow). Duplex ultrasound (*bottom row*) reveals a severe proximal stenosis of the right MCA with a maximal flow >3 m/s (left); findings in the left MCA are normal (right).

Diagnosis

Multiple cerebral infarctions in atherosclerotic middle cerebral artery stenosis.

General remarks

Atherosclerotic MCA stenosis is a less common occlusive disease in patients from western countries compared to those with asian ethnicity. In recent studies using DWI, three main patterns of cerebral infarcts were identified: (a) small subcortical lacunar-like infarcts, (b) border zone infarcts (anterior, posterior and internal border zone) and (c) cortical infarcts. Small subcortical infarcts are caused by both occlusion of the origin of a penetrating artery by an atheroma in the MCA or small embolic particles obstructing a penetrating artery. Border zone infarcts are most common as multiple chainlike infarcts and associated with more severe MCA-stenoses, therefore hemodynamic compromise is a possible mechanism for watershed-type infarcts. Cortical infarcts caused by MCA stenosis are usually small (less then 50 mm in diameter), but multiple, thus suggesting artery to artery embolism.

In many patients, like the one we present in this case, border zone and cortical infarct patterns are combined. This supports the hypothesis, put forward by

Caplan and Hennerici (1998) that hypoperfusion and embolism often coexist and may result in an impaired clearance of microemboli especially in the border zone regions.

Special remarks

Despite standard medical therapy with antiplatelet agents or oral anticoagulants, the risk of recurrent cerebral ischemic events in symptomatic MCA-stenoses is remarkably high with annual ipsilateral stroke rates of 9.5%. In contrast, medically treated asymptomatic MCA-stenoses appear to have a benign long-term prognosis.

Retrospective studies suggested a possible superiority of oral anticoagulants over antiplatelet agents in the secondary prophylaxis in patients with symptomatic intracranial stenosis (Kern *et al.*, 2005), but results from a prospective trial comparing both treatment strategies seems to favor aspirin (Chimowitz *et al.*, 2005).

SUGGESTED READING

Caplan, L. R. Intracranial branch atheromatous disease: a neglected, understudied and underused concept. *Neurology* 1989; **39**:1246–1250.

Caplan, L. R. & Hennerici, M. Impaired clearence of emboli (washout) is an important link between hypoperfusion, embolism and ischemic stroke. *Arch. Neurol.* 1998; **55**:1475–1482.

Chimowitz, M. I., Lynn, M. J., Howlett-Smith, H. *et al.* For the Warfarin–Aspirin Symptomatic Intracranial Disease Trial Investigators. Comparison of warfarin and aspirin for symptomatic intracranial arterial stenosis. *N. Engl. J. Med.* 2005; **352**:1305–1316.

Kern, R., Steinke, W., Daffertshofer, M., Prager, R., & Hennerici, M. Stroke recurrences in patients with symptomatic vs asymptomatic middle cerebral artery disease. *Neurology* 2005; **65**:859–864.

Lee, P. H., Oh, S. H., Bang, O. Y., Joo, S. Y., Joo, I. S., & Huh, K. Infarct patterns in artherosclerotic middle cerebral artery versus internal carotid artery disease. *Neurology* 2004; **62**:1291–1296.

Lyrer, P. A., Engelter, S., Radü, E. W., & Steck, A. J. Cerebral Infarcts related to isolated middle cerebral artery stenosis. *Stroke* 1997; **28**:1022–1027.

Sacco, R. L., Kargman, D. E., Gu, Q., & Zamanillo, M. C. Race-ethnicity and determinants of intracranial atherosclerotic cerebral infarction: the Northern Manhattan Stroke Study. *Stroke* 1995; **26**:14–20.

Wong, K. S., Gao, S., Chan, Y. L. *et al.* Mechanisms of acute cerebral infarctions in patients with middle cerebral artery stenosis: a diffusion-weighted imaging and microemboli monitoring study. *Ann. Neurol.* 2002; **52**:74–81.

Sudden weakness after holidays in Kenya

Clinical history

Two days after returning from a holiday in Kenya, a 32-year-old woman noticed sudden weakness of the left arm and leg. When after 6 hours her symptoms did not resolve, she came to the emergency room. Her health was excellent. She smoked cigarettes (20-pack–years) and took an oral contraceptive.

Examination

On admission, neurologic examination showed a slight sensorimotor hemiparesis on the left without any further neuropsychological deficits.

Neurological scores on admission
NIH 3; Barthel Index 95; GCS 15.

Special studies

Initial CT was normal, while MRI showed an acute infarct in the territory of the right middle cerebral artery. Cardiac examination revealed a mid-systolic murmur with a maximum at the second intercostal space on the left and a split S2. Thus, an atrial septal defect was suspected, which was confirmed by echo-cardiography. Compression ultrasound showed a thrombus in the deep veins of the left leg extending into the popliteal vein. All tests for coagulation ab-normalities, cerebrovascular ultrasound, and Holter ECG monitoring were normal.

Follow-up

Three weeks after admission, the atrial septal defect was closed by conventional surgery. The patient recovered well, and 2 months after the stroke, the patient had only a slight residual hemiparesis.

Image findings

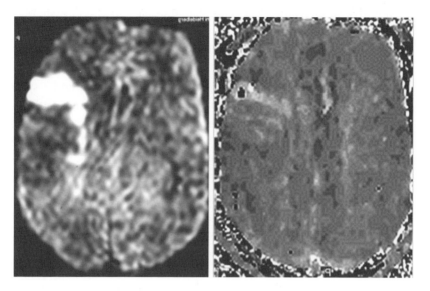

Figure 20.1 MRI on admission shows an acute infarct in the right MCA territory (DWI-weighted images, *left*) and a perfusion deficit that did not extend into the infarcted area (PWI-weighted images, *right*).

Diagnosis

Paradoxical embolus due to deep vein thrombosis and atrial septal defect, associated with a recent long-haul flight.

General remarks

In young patients (<50 years) with stroke, uncommon causes must be thoroughly investigated. Arterial dissection and cardiac embolism are the leading causes of stroke in this patient population. While a previously undiagnosed atrial septal defect is uncommon, it presents a condition which is easy to diagnose and warrants an aggressive treatment. This case also highlights the importance of the general physical examination in every stroke patient, because some diagnoses such as an atrial septal defect can be established with a high reliability using clinical findings alone.

Special remarks

Atrial septal defect (ASD) is the most frequent congenital heart defect, present in 4 out of 100 000 persons. If a patient has no other congenital defects, symptoms may be absent. Symptoms of ASD usually manifest by age 30. Individuals with ASD are at an increased risk of developing a number of complications including infective endocarditis, heart failure, and atrial fibrillation. Remarkably, cerebral embolism is a relatively rare event despite the obligatory shunt. In the majority of patients with ASD, characteristic findings upon cardiac auscultation are present. In the second or third intercostal space on the left, an early to midsytolic murmur can be heard. Typically, a fixed, widely split S2 and a systolic click or late systolic murmur at the apex is present. In patients with large shunts, auscultation at the lower left sternal border may reveal a low pitched diastolic murmur. These findings should be easily recognized even by neurologists who are not experts in cardiac auscultation. The diagnosis is usually confirmed by echocardiography. In contrast to the patent foramen ovale, where considerable uncertainties on the best management continue to exist, there is a broad consensus that patients with a large atrial septal defect or who are symptomatic are best treated by closure. The gold standard is surgical repair with sutures or grafts. However, in recent years, promising results have been published with endovascular devices that will likely eventually become the standard procedure in the near future.

There are several retrospective and a few prospective studies on venous thrombosis and PE after air travel. Although the comparability of these studies is limited, it can be concluded that there is a small risk of venous thrombosis following long-haul flights. The incidence of symptomatic DVT without PE is around 0.2%. The risk of clinically asymptomatic deep venous thrombosis lies around 1%. The data for short-range flights is scarce. Flights with a duration <6 hours likely carry no significantly increased risk of venous thrombosis. It is important, that in almost all persons with flight-associated venous thrombosis, additional predisposing risk factors are sought. In our patient, the combination of smoking and oral contraceptives is a well-known risk factor for venous thrombosis. There are only a few single case studies on stroke after air travel. Because of the frequency of both, air travel and stroke, in the general population, in the individual case, it is impossible to determine a causal relationship. However, a cardiac or pulmonary shunt has to be present to enable a paradoxical embolism from a venous thrombosis.

SUGGESTED READING

Attie, F., Rosas, M., Granados, N., Zabal, C., Buendía, A., & Calderón, J. Surgical treatment for secundum atrial septal defects in patients >40 years old. *J. Am. Coll. Cardiol.* 2001; **38**:2035–2042.

Dalen, J. E. Economy class syndrome *Arch. Intern. Med.* 2003; **163**:2674–2676.

Hughes, R. J., Hopkins, R. J., Hill, S. *et al.* Frequency of venous thromboembolism in low to moderate risk long distance air travellers: the New Zealand Air Traveller's Thrombosis (NZATT) study. *Lancet* 2003; **362**:2039–2044.

Konstantinides, S., Geibel, A., & Olschewski, M. A comparison of surgical and medical therapy in atrial septal defect in adults. *N. Engl. J. Med.* 1995; **333**:469–473.

Lapostolle, F., Borron, S. W., Surget, V., Sordelet, D., Lapandry, C., & Adnet F. Stroke associated with pulmonary embolism after air travel. *Neurology* 2003; **60**:1983–1985.

Martinelli, I., Taioli, E., Battaglioli, T. *et al.* Risk of venous thromboembolism after air travel. *Arch. Intern. Med.* 2003; **163**:2771–2774.

Rao, P. S. Catheter closure of atrial septal defects. *J. Invas. Cardiol.* 2003; **15**:398–400.

Schwarz, T., Siegert, G., Oettler, W. *et al.* Venous thrombosis following long-haul flights. *Arch. Intern. Med.* 2003; **163**:2759–2764.

Recurrent spells of right-sided weakness

Clinical history

A 56-year-old man suddenly developed dysarthria and a severe right-sided sensorimotor deficit. In the last 2 days before admission, seven very similar episodes had occurred, each one lasting between 5 to 20 minutes.

General history

Arterial hypertension, hyperhomocysteinemia, persistent foramen ovale.

Neurological scores

NIH 7; Barthel Index 90; GCS 15.

Examination

On admission the patient presented with right sensory motor hemiparesis and dysarthria. The patient received i.v. tissue plasminogen activator treatment, followed by i.v. heparin. Cranial CT and MRI scans were normal. The patient was free of symptoms on discharge and secondary prevention was started with aspirin (300 mg/day). Two months later, the patient presented again with a very similar clinical picture. Over 3 days, repeated stereotyped TIAs consisting of dysarthria and right limb weakness reoccurred: 7 episodes on day 1, 20 episodes on day 2 and 10 TIAs on day 3 that lasted for 5 to 20 minutes as observed during his first hospital stay. On day 4, a permanent deficit developed with right-sided hemiparesis including the face and dysarthria.

Neurological scores:

Date	First hospitalization			Second hospitalization		
	NIH	Barthel index	Ranking scale	NIH	Barthel index	Ranking scale
First day	7	90	2	7	90	2
Discharge	0	100	0	5	90	1

Special studies

MRI including diffusion-weighted imaging was performed on the first and seventh day of the second hospital stay and finally revealed a lacunar infarction in the left pons.

Image findings

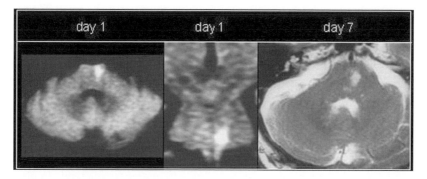

Figure 21.1 Diffusion-weighted MR images (*left, middle*) and T$_2$-weighted image (*right*) taken during the second hospitalisation of the patient. Left pontine infarction is shown in transverse (*left, right*) and coronal plane (*middle*).

Diagnosis

Repeat pontine warning syndrome.

General remarks

The CWS, also known as Donnan syndrome, describes transient neurological signs that occur in a stereotyped repetitive manner up to several days, mostly followed by persistent deficits and imaging signs of lacunar infarction. They represent a particular form of TIAs, which are often a "warning sign" for an impending brain infarction and are often a "warning sign" for pending cerebral infarction and could be attributed to lesions in the internal capsule. In the Harvard Stroke registry emphasis was placed on the presence of TIAs preceding lacunar infarction. The TIAs were usually stereotyped and brief and might repeat many times during one to 3 days. The "capsular warning syndrome" was named by Donnan in 1987. His patient presented with a hemiplegia caused by cerebral infarction in the posterior part of the internal capsule. Pathology of penetrating arteries was assumed to cause the brief episodes of often dramatic deficits with intermittent complete resolution. However, pontine lesions may also cause this clinically important syndrome.

Special remarks

Our case presented twice with very similar clinical deficits pointing to a particular brain area the function of which had been repeatedly disturbed. While the first presentation did not result in infarction, the second cluster of TIAs was followed by a lasting deficit and MR findings consistent with a lacunar pontine infarct. Despite the fact that a patent foramen ovale was found by echocardiography, we propose a microangiopathic origin of the symptoms as the most likely cause. Interestingly, during the first cluster of TIAs thrombolytic therapy led to a complete and lasting resolution of symptoms. As described by others, we were unable to prevent TIAs by i.v. heparin treatment during the second cluster of symptoms. This clinical condition is a challenge for new therapeutic measures to prevent imminent infarction. Some have advocated keeping the patient recumbent and liberally administering fluids to augment collateral circulation.

Currently, the fluctuating pattern of severe deficits is not well understood. The usual explanation is blockage of a penetrating artery with tenuous collateral supply that is decompensated by hemorrheological changes in the circulation (altered blood pressure, blood volume, or whole blood viscosity). Intermittent spreading depression-like depolarizations that are triggered by ischemic foci is another explanation that accounts for the high frequency of symptomatic intervals, their stereotyped appearance and their fate in terms of final infarction. By contrast, other potential causes such as vasospasm or cardiac/arterial sources of emboli, are unable to explain all features of the case presented.

SUGGESTED READING

Benito-Leon, J., Alvarez-Linera, J., & Porta-Etessam, J. Detection of acute pontine infarction by diffusion-weighted MRI in capsular warning syndrome. *Cerebrovasc. Dis.* 2001; **11**:350–351.

Donnan, G. A. & Bladin, P. F. The capsular warning syndrome: repetitive hemiplegic events preceding capsular stroke. *Stroke* 1987; **18**:296.

Donnan, G. A., O'Malley, H. M., Quang, L., Hurley, S., & Bladin, P. F. The capsular warning syndrome: pathogenesis and clinical features. *Neurology* 1993; **43**:957–962.

Farrar, J. & Donnan, G. A. Capsular warning syndrome preceding pontine infarction. *Stroke* 1993; **24**:762.

Mohr, J. P., Caplan, L. R., Malski, J. W. *et al.* The Harvard Cooperative Stroke registry: a prospective registry. *Neurology* 1978; **28**:754–762.

Staaf, G., Geijer, B., Lindgren, A., & Norrving, B. Diffusion-weighted MRI findings in patients with capsular warning syndrome. *Cerebrovasc. Dis.* 2004; **17**:1–8.

An uncommon cause of CVT

Clinical history

A 27-year-old woman was hospitalized after a first generalized epileptic seizure preceded by a severe headache during the previous 2 days. She had been taking oral contraceptives during the preceding 4 months, did not smoke and had no signs of infection. At the age of 4, dislocated ocular lenses were removed by operation. Further medical history was unrevealing. There were no family members with known premature vascular disease.

Examination

Neurological examination of this agitated patient showed a slight left hemiparesis. Cognitive and sensory functions were normal.

Special studies

An MRI scan showed incomplete thrombosis of the superior sagittal sinus without any abnormalities in the brain parenchyma. She was treated with anticoagulants and antiepileptic drugs, and rapidly recovered. On MRI follow-up, the thrombosis had partly recanalized. Laboratory testing revealed an elevated homocysteine blood level of 167 µmol/l (normal <13 µmol/l). The patient was found to be a heterozygous carrier of the methylene-tetrahydrofolate-reductase (MTHFR) C667T mutation associated with hyperhomocysteinemia. She was given vitamin B_{12} and folate. As low titer antiphospholipid antibodies was also present, suspicion of an antiphospholipid-antibody syndrome was raised, which possibly contributed to the dural sinus thrombosis. Oral anticoagulants were continued.

Follow-up

On follow-up 1 year later, the patient reported pain in the right hip. X-ray and bone density measures revealed signs of osteoporosis. By that time, antiphospholipid antibodies were no longer detectable, whereas the homocysteine level was still high (209 µmol/l). Tests of other amino acid levels showed hypermethionemia (510 μmol/l, normal range 15–32) and low cysteine levels (16 μmol/l, normal range 31–50). This confirmed the diagnosis of classical homocystinuria, further supported by two heterozygous mutations in the cystathionine beta synthetase gene. Patients with homocystinuria often have Marfan-like features. High dose supplementation with pyridoxine (1000 mg daily) did not cause a decrease of homocysteine levels so that a methionine-depleted diet was begun. Within 3 months, homocysteine levels dropped to 44 μmol/l. Oral anticoagulants were then replaced by 100 mg aspirin.

Image findings

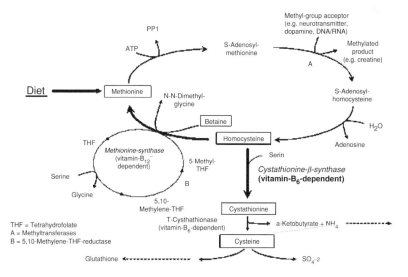

Figure 22.1 MR phlebography (*on the left*) and T_2-weighted coronal section showing the lack of flow (black arrows) and the thrombus (white arrow) in the superior sagittal sinus.

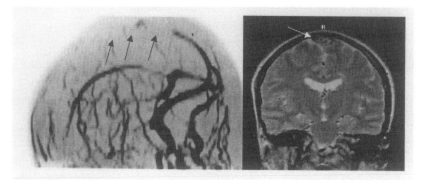

Figure 22.2 Homocysteine metabolism (from Stanger *et al.*, 2003).

Diagnosis

Thrombosis of superior sagittal sinus in a patient with homocystinuria.

General remarks

Hyperhomocysteinemia is a known risk factor for vascular disease. The prevalence of moderate hyperhomocysteinemia (13 to 30 μmol/l) is about 5%–10% in the general population, and even this slight elevation seems to increase the risk of CVT. The elevation is correlated with the methylene-tetrahydrofolate-reductase C667T mutation, for which our patient is heterozygous. However, her homocysteine level was about 200 μmol/l. Blood levels exceeding 100 μmol/l indicate classical homocystinuria. This hereditary metabolic disorder of an estimated prevalence of 1:344 000 worldwide is most commonly caused by one of several known mutations in the CBS gene, two of which were found in our patient. This enzyme catalyzes the synthesis of cysthationine from homocysteine and serine in a pyridoxine (vitamin B$_6$)-dependent pathway. In CBS deficiency, elevated levels of homocysteine and methionine, as well as low cysteine levels, are found. In homozygous carriers of this mutation, homocysteine blood levels of up to 50 times higher than normal are found, whereas heterozygotes seem not to have elevated levels.

Special remarks

There are very few cases of cerebral venous thrombosis in homocystinuria, some are described in childhood. However, Linnebank and coworkers screened 46 adult patients with CVT for the most common CBS gene mutation (I278T) and found one homozygous carrier with previously undiagnosed homocystinuria. As homocystinuria is rare, the diagnosis is often delayed. In pyridoxine-responsive forms of CBS deficiency, a near normal homocysteine level can be achieved by supplementing pyridoxine. In pyridoxine non-responsive forms, a significant lowering of the homocysteine level can still be realized by adding betaine, an alternative methyl-donator, resulting in remethylation of homocysteine, and by implementing a methionine-depleted diet. If patients remain untreated, vascular thrombotic events occur before the age of 30 in half of the affected patients.

FIRST DESCRIPTION

Carson, N. A., Cusworth, D. C., Dent, C. E., Field, C. M., Neill, D. W., & Westall, R. G. Homocystinuria: a new inborn error of metabolism associated with mental deficiency. *Arch. Dis. Child.* 1963; **38**:425–436.

CURRENT REVIEW

Linnebank, M., Junker, R., Nabavi, D. G., Linnebank, A., & Koch, H. G. Isolated thrombosis due to the cystathionine beta-synthase mutation c.833T>C (1278T). *J. Inherit. Metab. Dis.* 2003; **26**:509–511.

Stanger, O., Herrmann, W., Pietrzik, K. *et al.* DACH-LIGA homocystein (German, Austrian and Swiss Homocysteine Society): consensus paper on the rational clinical use of homocysteine, folic acid and B-vitamins in cardiovascular and thrombotic diseases: guidelines and recommendations. *Clin. Chem. Lab. Med.* 2003; **41**:1392–1403.

Yap, S., Boers, G. H., Wilcken, B. *et al.* Vascular outcome in patients with homocystinuria due to cystathionine beta-synthase deficiency treated chronically: a multicenter observational study. *Arterioscler. Thromb. Vasc. Biol.* 2001; **21**:2080–2085.

SUGGESTED READING

Buoni, S., Molinelli, M., Mariottini, A. *et al.* Homocystinuria with transverse sinus thrombosis. *J. Child. Neurol.* 2001; **16**:688–690.

Cochran, F. B. & Packman, S. Homocystinuria presenting as sagittal sinus thrombosis. *Eur. Neurol.* 1992; **32**:1–3.

Case 23

"My arm no longer belongs to me. . ."

Clinical history

Three days and again 24 hours prior to her admission, the 78-year-old woman had two episodes of sudden numbness of her left arm accompanied by a strange feeling that the arm no longer belonged to her, lasting for about 15 minutes. On the morning of admission, the numbness and feeling of an alien presence of her left arm recurred, this time accompanied by purposeless movements of the arm that seemed to be under external, extravolitional control. She felt urged to talk to her hand "you don't have to help me" when performing movements with the right hand. The patient did not recognize any paresis of the left arm. These symptoms persisted for 5 hours; however, the patient presented to the emergency unit just after complete remission.

General history

Hypercholesterolemia, arterial hypertension.

Examination

General examination was abnormal for a blood pressure of 170/90 mmHg. Examination of cranial nerves, motor function, coordination and extensive sensory testing was normal apart from mild action tremor of the right hand. The patient was right-handed. Her deep tendon reflexes were symmetrical and normal; there was a flexor plantar response.

Special studies

Emergency CT excluded intracranial bleeding and was otherwise inconclusive. Twenty-four hours later, MR DWI of the brain showed a small acute hyperintense lesion in the hand area of the right postcentral gyrus, in addition there were small hyperintense lesions in the left parietooccipital cortex and subcortical white matter in the area of the posterior borderzone between the PCA and MCA territories. MRA revealed a reduced flow signal in the left ICA. MR PWI showed a delayed perfusion of the left MCA territory in time to peak maps. Extracranial Doppler and duplex sonography demonstrated a left 90% ICA stenosis, and transcranial Doppler sonography was suggestive of collateral flow via the ACA and ACoA from the right to the left side. Cardiac investigations showed no source of embolism and blood laboratory values including coagulation studies were completely normal. For secondary stroke prevention, platelet aggregation inhibition was changed from daily aspirin 50 mg/d to twice daily aspirin 25 mg/ extended release dipyridamol 200 mg. The patient refused to undergo carotid endarterectomy on the left. She was counseled for treatment of her cerebrovascular risk factors.

Image findings

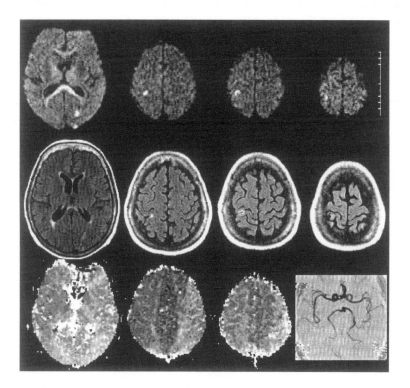

Figure 23.1 Small infarct in the right postcentral sensory cortex/subcortex. Small cortical and deep borderzone infarct in the left MCA/PCA borderzone (MRI, DWI – top row; FLAIR – *middle row*). Time-to-peak PWI showing delayed bolus arrival in the left MCA territory (*bottom row*). Intracranial MRA with reduced signal intensity in projection onto the left ICA and MCA branches on the left (*bottom row, far right*).

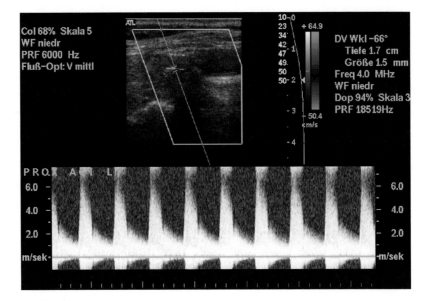

Figure 23.2 Color-coded duplex sonography and pulsed-wave Doppler sonography of left proximal internal carotid artery revealing high-grade (90%) ICA stenosis.

Diagnosis

Transient posterior type alien limb syndrome on the left due to right sensory cortex/subcortex infarction, additional asymptomatic left MCA/PCA border zone infarction in the presence of a 90% left ICA stenosis.

General remarks

The alien limb phenomenon or alien hand sign is a rare presentation of cerebral ischemia. If present, this syndrome can be mostly observed in the acute phase of ischemia, lasting for minutes up to a few days, but it may occasionally persist for months. Other causes of the alien hand syndrome include tumors, intracerebral bleedings, ruptured aneurysms – mostly of the ACA and often with surgical clipping – callosotomy for epilepsy, and neurodegenerative disorders such as corticobasal degeneration. The first description of the alien hand phenomenon was by Kurt Goldstein (1908), and in his patient there was infarction of the anterior corpus callosum and the right hemisphere due to ACA infarction. The term "la main étrangère" was coined by Brion and Jedynak in 1972. Originally, the alien hand syndrome was described as a consequence of callosal or medial frontal lobe damage, and in their review, Feinberg *et al.* (1992) tried to correlate distinct clinical patterns to a callosal and a frontal subtype of alien hand syndrome. In the callosal type, damage to the corpus callosum with or without the right or bilateral frontal lobes was observed, the nondominant hand was affected, and the patients presented with intermanual conflict and less often grasping or compulsory tool manipulation. In the frontal type, the damage was in the left medial frontal lobe and corpus callosum, the dominant hand was affected, and the patients showed grasping and compulsory tool manipulation and rarely intermanual conflicts. In recent years, a posterior type of alien hand syndrome has been added, when damage to the lateral thalamus, parietal cortex and subcortex, and the temporal lobe was described. The patients reported feelings of the arm wandering, instances of levitation, purposeless arm movements and foreignness of the arm. In parietal lesions, neglect of several sensory modalities were also found. There are now several cases of alien limb syndrome displaying well documented posterior pathology without involvement of the frontal lobes or the corpus callosum, including a case of damage in the pre-/postcentral gyri similar to our patient, thus the recognition of the existence of a posterior subtype of alien limb syndrome seems justified.

Special remarks

The patient presented with recurrent transient ischemic attacks, that were remarkable for the manifestation of an alien hand sign in the non-dominant hand. Moreover, there were unsuspected bilateral cerebral infarcts. The distribution of the simultaneous lesions suggested an emboligenic origin, however a source of embolism was not detected. The situation was complicated by a high-grade ICA stenosis on the left and indeed the ischemia of the left hemisphere was located in the MCA/PCA borderzone. Caplan and Hennerici (1998) hypothesized that infarction due to embolism should occur in this area because of "reduced emboli washout" due to relative hypoperfusion. Our case snuggly fits this concept. It remains debatable whether the infarction in the left hemisphere had occurred asymptomatically as the patient had not reported any corresponding neurological dysfunction, nor would it have been mandatory for the alien limb syndrome. Considering the new data of the ACST trial referring to an operative benefit in asymptomatic high-grade carotid stenosis and the additional imaging evidence of recent subcortical ischemia in the left carotid territory, an endarterectomy seemed warranted; however, this was declined by the patient.

FIRST DESCRIPTION

Brion, S. & Jedynak, C. P. Troubles du transfert interhemisphérique. A propos de trois observations de tumeurs du corps calleux. Le signe de la main étrangère. *Rev. Neurol. (Paris)* 1972; **126**:257–266.

Goldstein, K. Zur Lehre der motorischen Apraxie. *J. Psychol. Neurol.* 1908; **11**:169–187.

CURRENT REVIEW

Fisher, C. M. Alien hand phenomena: a review with the addition of six personal cases. *Can. J. Neurol. Sci.* 2000; **27**:192–203.

Scepkowski, L. A. & Cronin-Golomb, A. The alien hand: cases, categorizations, and anatomical correlates. *Behav. Cogn. Neurosci. Rev.* 2003; **2**:261–277.

SUGGESTED READING

Andre, C. & Domingues, R. C. Transient alien hand syndrome: is this a seizure or a transient ischaemic attack? *J. Neurol. Neurosurg. Psychiatry* 1996; **60**:232–233.

Bundick, T. & Spinella, M. Subjective experience, involuntary movement, and posterior alien hand syndrome. *J. Neurol. Neurosurg. Psychiatry* 2000; **68**:83–85.

Caplan, L. R. & Hennerici, M. Impaired clearance of emboli (washout) is an important link between hypoperfusion, embolism, and ischemic stroke. *Arch. Neurol.* 1998; **55**:1475–1482.

Feinberg, T. E., Schindler, R. J., Flanagan, N. G., & Haber, L. D. Two alien hand syndromes. *Neurology* 1992; **42**:19–24.

MRC Asymptomatic Carotid Surgery Trial (ACST) Collaborative Group. Prevention of disabling and fatal strokes by successful carotid endarterectomy in patients without recent neurological symptoms: randomised controlled trial. *Lancet* 2004; **363**: 1491–1502.

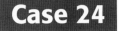

Coma of unknown onset in an old lady

Clinical history

A 76-year-old woman presented to our emergency room with coma of unknown onset. The referring emergency physician scored the patient with 7 points on the Glasgow Coma Scale. She had normal pupils, reacting equally to light. Because of a worsening respiratory state, the patient was intubated and mechanically ventilated before transporting her to our hospital.

General history

Her family physician had treated her in the past for long-standing history of hypertension, coronary heart disease, and atrial fibrillation.

Examination

On admission, her blood pressure was 190/100mmHg, HR 54, heartbeat rhythmical. She was comatous, intubated, mechanically ventilated, treated with sedatives and muscle relaxants. Pupils were both 1.5mm, not reacting to light, corneal reflexes were missing. There was no reaction on painful stimuli, manipulation of the tracheal tube elicited a weak cough – MRI studies were impossible under these circumstances.

Neurological scores on admission

NIH 36; Barthel Index 0; GCS 7.

Special studies

Initial CT scans were normal, with the exception of a questionable hyperdense MCA sign on the right. Conventional cerebral angiography – performed to identify and potentially treat basilar artery thrombosis – showed an occlusion of the MCA stem on the right and a M2-segment occlusion of the left MCA. Systemic thrombolysis – rather than bilateral intraarterial – with 75mg rtPA was started 90 minutes after arrival at our hospital. Follow-up CT, performed 60 minutes after finishing thrombolysis revealed early signs of infarction in the complete right MCA territory. The following day, her clinical condition was unchanged. Follow-up angiography revealed recanalization of a single MCA branch on the right and recanalization of the occluded M2-segment on the left. With further clinical deterioration and loss of caudal brainstem reflexes, a third CT scan showed a malignant complete MCA infarction on the right side and a temporoparietal 1/3 MCA infarction with hemorrhagic transformation on the left. The patient died the same day due to generalized brain edema secondary to malignant bilateral MCA territory infarctions.

On pathological examination, besides multiple pulmonary embolism, deep venous thromboses in muscular veins of both calves could be proven. A large patent foramen ovale was present. Signs of elevated pulmonary pressure were detected with enlarged right ventricle, congestion of liver and spleen. In the right MCA a residual thrombus was detected, which was identical on histological examination compared to thrombotic material in the deep muscular calf veins (coagulation thrombus). No thrombus was shown in the left MCA. Severe brain edema with signs of brain herniation were present.

Image findings

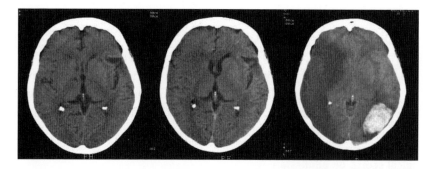

Figure 24.1 Initial CT scans were unremarkable (left) Follow-up CT, performed 60 minutes after finishing systemic thrombolysis revealed early signs of infarction in the complete right MCA territory (middle). With further clinical deterioration and loss of caudal brainstem reflexes, a third CT-scan showed a malignant complete MCA infarction on the right side and a temporoparietal 1/3 MCA infarction with hemorrhagic transformation on the left (right).

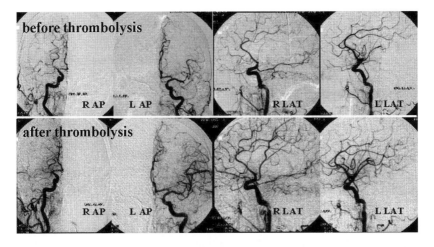

Figure 24.2 In the conventional angiography on admission, an occlusion of the MCA stem on the right and a M2-segment occlusion of the left MCA were diagnosed (upper row, from left to right: right anterior–posterior internal carotid angiogram, left anterior–posterior internal carotid angiogram, right lateral internal carotid angiogram, left lateral internal carotid angiogram). Systemic thrombolysis with 75 mg rtPA was performed 90 minutes after arrival at our hospital. The follow-up angiography immediately after systemic thrombolysis revealed recanalisation of a single MCA branch on the right and recanalisation of the occluded M2-segment on the left (lower row, from left to right: right anterior–posterior internal carotid angiogram, left anterior–posterior internal carotid angiogram, right lateral internal carotid angiogram, left lateral internal carotid angiogram).

Diagnosis

Bilateral simultaneous MCA infarction due to paradoxical embolism on the basis of bilateral deep venous thromboses.

General remarks

In this patient, bihemispheric large MCA infarctions occurred simultaneously, which is certainly a very rare condition. The chain of causation for this rare event is complete in this case, since presumably multiple thromboses in deep muscular calf veins led to repeated PE with a consecutive rise in right atrial pressure with subsequent paradoxical embolism via a large PFO. Other potential cardiac sources of systemic embolism such as left atrial large thrombi, atrial myxoma, or endocarditis may cause simultaneous or closely sequential strokes in multiple territories, although the reported cases often show small infarcts in multiple territories.

The high frequency (35%) of PFO in patients with major PE has been reported and is in accord with autopsy findings from the Mayo Clinic. Right-to-left shunting via a PFO does not occur under normal conditions unless right atrial pressure exceeds that in the left atrium. With right ventricular dilatation after PE, right atrial pressure rises and right-to-left shunt ensues via the PFO. Such a shunting not only causes arterial desaturation and thus systemic hypoxemia but also paradoxic embolism in either the cerebral or the coronary circulation, either or both of which may result in serious consequences. Therefore, in cases with venous thromboembolism and raised right heart pressures, a patent foramen ovale may permit paradoxical emboli, which could complicate the course of patients with PE. Few cases are published showing a thrombus trapped in a PFO, a condition called impending paradoxical embolism. In the case of a young man reported by Claver *et al.*, the patient was in coma because of a traffic accident, then had first a pulmonary embolus followed immediately afterwards by a cerebral embolus. Transesophageal echocardiography revealed a giant thrombus trapped in foramen ovale protruding to the right and left ventricles. Chow and colleagues, while reviewing the English literature during the past 20 years, identified 60 reported cases of impending paradoxical embolism. They recommend that patients with impending paradoxical embolism be treated with initial systemic heparinization followed by emergent surgical embolectomy if the surgical risks are acceptable.

Special remarks

In our patient, the unusual diagnosis of bilateral simultaneous MCA embolism was made by conventional angiography. Given the fact that the prognosis with simultaneous bihemispheric territorial infarctions was unfavorable, and no infarct demarcation on CT was seen, systemic thrombolysis was performed even though the exact symptom onset was unknown. Follow-up angiography disclosed partial bilateral recanalization of the severe embolic process. This may be due in part to the fact that emboli arising from the venous system are more susceptible to thrombolytic agents such as rtPA compared to thrombi originating from arterial sources. Unfortunately, recanalization occurred too late and malignant MCA infarction on the right with hemorrhagic transformation of left hemispheric stroke finally led to death 24 hours after intervention.

FIRST DESCRIPTION

Cohnheim, J. Thrombose & Embolie. In *Vorlesungen Über Allgemeine Pathologie*. Berlin, Germany: Hirschwald, 1877; 134.

CURRENT REVIEW

Lamy, C., Giannesini, C., Zuber, M. *et al.* Clinical and imaging findings in cryptogenic stroke patients with and without patent foramen ovale: the PFO-ASA Study. Atrial Septal Aneurysm. *Stroke* 2002; **33**:706–711.

SUGGESTED READING

Arquizan, C., Lamy, C., & Mas, J. L. Infarctus cérébraux multiples simultanés sustentoriels. *Rev. Neurol. (Paris)* 1997; **153**:748–753.

Chartier, L., Bera, J., Delomez, M. *et al.* Free-floating thrombi in the right heart: diagnosis, management, and prognostic indexes in 38 consecutive patients. *Circulation* 1999; **99**:2779–2783.

Chow, B. J., Johnson, C. B., Turek, M., & Burwash, I. G. Impending paradoxical embolus: a case report and review of the literature. *Can. J. Cardiol.* 2003; **19**:1426–1432.

Claver, E., Larrousse, E., Bernal, E., Lopez-Ayerbe, J., & Valle, V. Giant thrombus trapped in foramen ovale with pulmonary embolus and stroke. *J. Am. Soc. Echocardiogr.* 2004; **17**:916–918.

Hagen, P. T., Scholz, D. G., & Edwards, W. D. Incidence and size of patent foramen ovale during the first 10 decades of life: an autopsy study of 965 normal hearts. *Mayo Clin. Proc.* 1984; **59**:17–20.

Konstantinides, S., Geibel, A., Kasper, W., Olschewski, M., Blümel, L., & Just, H. Patent foramen ovale is an important predictor of adverse outcome in patients with major pulmonary embolism. *Circulation* 1998; **97**:1946–1951.

Szabo, K., Kern, R., Gass, A., Hirsch, J., & Hennerici, M. Acute stroke patterns in patients with internal carotid artery disease: a diffusion-weighted magnetic resonance imaging study. *Stroke* 2001; **32**:1323–1329.

Case 25

Spreading sensation of the left arm and face

Clinical history

A 73-year-old man noticed recurrent stereotypic spells with numbness of his left hand, spreading over his forearm and shoulder to the left side of his face, and resolving completely after a maximum of 15 minutes. These episodes occurred about once a day for several days and were not accompanied by headache or any further neurological symptoms.

General history

Arterial hypertension, diabetes mellitus type 2.

Examination

The findings on neurological examination were normal.

Neurological scores

NIH 0; Barthel Index 100; GCS 15.

Special studies

A right parietal theta-focus on electroencephalography affirmed the clinically suspected simple partial sensory seizures with Jacksonian march. Computed tomography and MRI revealed subarachnoid hemorrhage in the right central sulcus and a localized intracerebral hemorrhage in the postcentral gyrus. Magnetic resonance venography as well as conventional angiography displayed all cortical and dural veins as normal. A predisposing factor known to be associated with venous thrombosis could not be identified. The patient received anticonvulsive therapy; however, due to the lack of a persistent occlusive pathology or prothrombotic tendencies, no anticoagulant medication was initiated.

Follow-up

The patient remained seizure-free with antiepileptic medication. A follow-up MRI after 8 weeks showed residual subarachnoid blood still detectable in the central sulcus.

Image findings

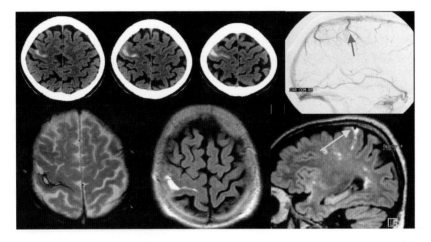

Figure 25.1 Native CT showing intraparenchymal and subarachnoid hemorrhage in the postcentral gyrus and central sulcus (upper row, three images from left side). DSA after contrast agent application to the right carotid artery (upper row, right). All right-hemispheric cortical veins are depicted easily. Red arrow points to the vein in the central sulcus. Hypodense susceptibility artifact in T_2^*-weighted images (lower row, left). Hyperdense signal in FLAIR (lower row, middle). Perpendicular view of the cortical vein (yellow arrow) in the central sulcus, flow void is visible (lower row, right). The depth of the sulcus is filled with blood.

Diagnosis

Isolated cortical vein thrombosis with subarachnoid hemorrhage.

General remarks

The term cerebral venous thrombosis most often refers to thrombosis of one of the major dural sinuses. Isolated involvement of a cortical vein especially without sinus involvement is rare and predominantly described in case reports. Clinical diagnosis can be difficult as clinical manifestation may range from headache only in about one-half of the patients, to partial seizures and persisting focal neurological symptoms, such as aphasia, hemiparesis, agraphia, dyslexia and hemianopia. In the past, conventional angiography was regarded as the gold standard for the diagnosis of cerebral venous thrombosis. With the advent of MR imaging, however, with typical appearance of the clot in different stages, conventional angiography is now rarely required for diagnosis.

Special remarks

SAH is a rare presentation of cerebral venous thrombosis. The symptoms in our patient are likely to be related to the irritative effects of SAH around the central sulcus. We postulate that SAH was caused by isolated thrombosis of a cortical vein, probably the vein of Trolard. A direct visualization of thrombotic material or absence of flow, flow void and contrast agent in the affected vein was not possible. We interpreted this as a spontaneous recanalization of the parietal vein. Given the dynamic nature of venous thrombosis and the knowledge of the time course of signal intensity changes, it may well be that in some cases thrombus visualization is not possible due to fast recanalization, especially if small venous structures are affected.

FIRST DESCRIPTION

Raymond, F. Thrombose des veines parietales: ramollissement cerebral aigu. Aphasie. Contractures. Gazette des Hôpitaux; 1880; 1066.

CURRENT REVIEW

Jacobs, K., Moulin, T. Bogousslavsky, J. *et al.* The stroke syndrome of cortical vein thrombosis: *Neurology* 1996; **47**:376–382.

SUGGESTED READING

Ahn, T. B. & Roh, J. K. A case of cortical vein thrombosis with the cord sign: *Arch. Neurol.* 2003; **60**:1314–1316.

Ameri, A. & Bousser, M. G. Cerebral venous thrombosis. *Neurol. Clin.* 1992; **10**:87–111.

Chang, R. & Friedman, D. P. Isolated cortical venous thrombosis presenting as sub-arachnoid hemorrhage: a report of three cases. *Am. J. Neuroradiol.* 2004; **25**:1676–1679.

Tang, O. S., Ng, E. H., Wai, C. P., & Chung, H. P. Cortical vein thrombosis misinterpreted as intracranial haemorrhage in severe ovarian hyperstimulation syndrome: case report. *Hum. Reprod.* 2000; **15**:1913–1916.

Vuillier, F., Moulin, T. Tatu, L. Rumbach, L., & Bertrand, M. A. Isolated cortical vein thrombosis and activated protein C resistance. *Stroke* 1996; **27**:1440–1441.

From dysarthria to locked-in syndrome

Clinical history

An 83-year-old right-handed man was admitted after the acute onset of dysarthria, dysphagia and severe right hemiparesis. His past medical history was positive for the risk factors hypertension and non-insulin dependent diabetes mellitus. Medication consisted of 100 mg aspirin and 10 mg enalapril per day.

Neurological scores
NIH 10; Barthel Index 65; GCS 15.

Special studies

MRI showed a left paramedian infarction of the pons. Both MRA and transcranial Doppler ultrasound revealed a moderate stenosis of the proximal basilar artery extending over a distance of approximately 1 cm.

Despite anticoagulant treatment with heparin, the patient developed progressive loss of consciousness and quadriplegia on the fourth day of hospitalization. Repeat MRI now showed contralateral acute ischemia of the pons directly located cranially from the previous left-sided infarction. The degree of basilar artery stenosis on MRA remained unchanged.

Follow-up

During the next 7 days, the clinical status of the patient remained unchanged. He was comatose, quadriplegic with bilaterally positive Babinski's signs, and showed only mild undirected defense reaction to pain stimuli, but was breathing spontaneously. Then, however, the level of consciousness slowly improved. Four weeks after admission, he achieved a status in which he was awake for some hours during the day, but unable to phonate, to swallow, or to perform any voluntary movement of his limbs. However, he was now able to communicate with his eye muscles and the lid openers, which were the only muscles allowing voluntary movements.

Neurological scores
NIH 33; Barthel Index 5; GCS 6.

Follow-up 2

The condition of a locked-in syndrome, enabling the patient to communicate via voluntary eye and lid movements for a few hours during the day, continued for a period of 9 days. Then he again developed coma that was later complicated by febrile pulmonary infection. Six weeks after admission, the patient died due to progressive sepsis and renal failure.

Image findings

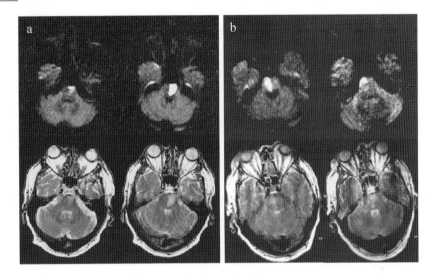

Figure 26.1 MRI on admission. (a) Diffusion-weighted imaging demonstrates an acute large brainstem infarction located in the left paramedian section of the pons. (b) Four days later, a contralateral acute ischemia of the pons was detected.

Diagnosis

Locked-in syndrome evoked by consecutive bilateral infarction of the pons.

General remarks

Locked-in syndrome is caused by the disruption of corticobulbar and cortico-spinal pathways. It is defined by sustained eye opening, awareness of the environment, aphonia or hypophonia, quadriplegia or quadriparesis, and vertical or lateral eye movement or blinking of the upper eyelid to signal yes/no responses. Eye or eyelid movements are the main method of communication.

In 1876, Darolles described a 30-year-old woman who developed a locked-in syndrome due to acute basilar artery occlusion. Typical "locked-in" features were present for a few hours until the death of the patient. The term "locked-in syndrome" was first used in 1966 by Plum and Posner.

Special remarks

Locked in syndrome is most commonly (approximately 75%) caused by cerebro-vascular disease. Other causes may be trauma, encephalitis or pontine myelino-lysis. Recent positron emission tomography (PET) studies have shown that cortical areas of patients in a locked-in syndrome have a comparable metabolism to normal controls. These findings emphasize that it is very important to make the diagnosis quickly and recognize the situation of the patient with awareness of self and environment in immobile bodies. Depending on age, concomitant disease and medical care, life expectancy may be several decades. Novel approaches to computer-based communication methods have substantially improved the quality of life in such chronic cases.

SUGGESTED READING

American Congress of Rehabilitation Medicine. Recommendation for use of uniform nomenclature pertinent to patients with severe alterations of consciousness. *Arch. Phys. Med. Rehabil.* 1995; **76**:205–209.

Kübler A., Wolpaw J. R., & Birbaumer N. Brain–computer communication: unlocking the locked in. *Psychol Bull.* 2001; **3**:358–375.

Laureys, S., Owen, A. M., & Schiff, N. D. Brain function in coma, vegetative state, and related disorders. *Lancet Neurol.* 2004; **3**:537–546. (Review).

Patterson, J. R. & Grabois, M. Locked-in syndrome: a review of 139 cases. *Stroke* 1986; **17**:758–764.

Plum, F. & Posner, J. B. *The Diagnosis of Stupor and Coma.* 3rd edn. Philadelphia: F. A. Davis, 1983.

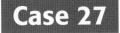

The woman who could not smile on command

Clinical history

A 48-year-old woman presented with acute onset of slight sensory–motor hemi-paresis of the right side with fast remission within 2 hours, leaving a residual facial asymmetry and slight pyramidal weakness (pronator drift) of the right arm. Previous medical history was unrevealing. Initial computed tomography of the brain was normal; duplex ultrasound of extra- and intracranial vessels showed plaques in both internal carotid arteries without significant stenosis. On the third day of hospitalization she suddenly lost the ability to speak.

Examination

On neurological examination she was awake and alert, anarthric with bilateral loss of voluntary control over muscles supplied by the cranial nerves V, VII, IX, X and XII in addition to the residual slight brachio-facial paresis on the right side. She understood spoken and written language, but was unable to speak. "Automatic voluntary dissociation" was observed with preserved ability to cry and smile but no voluntary control over muscles of face, jaw, tongue, and pharynx. Neuropsychological testing showed no impairment of comprehension, writing or reading. She was unable to swallow on command but reflex swallowing was well preserved. Gag reflex was diminished bilaterally. There was no sign of additional new motor or sensory deficit.

Neurological scores
NIH 4; Barthel Index 95; GCS 15.

Special studies

Emergency MRI using a stroke protocol was performed within 40 minutes after onset of acute anarthria: DWI and T_2-weighted images demonstrated the lesion in the left precentral region responsible for the initial clinical symptoms and hospi-talization. In addition, DWI showed a faint hyperintense stroke lesion in evolution in frontal and temporal cortical regions of the right MCA territory involving the anterior and posterior operculum 40 minutes after symptom onset, that was confirmed by a marked perfusion deficit in the corresponding area on PWI in the distribution of the prerolandic branch of the MCA.

The stroke evaluation showed a patent foramen ovale as a possible mechanism of paradoxical cerebral embolism.

Follow-up

Over the next 8 days the patient made a gradual recovery with marked improvement of oro-facial motor and speech functions.

Image findings

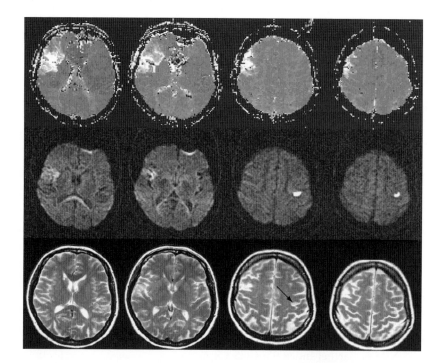

Figure 27.1 (*Top*) Perfusion studies with time-to-peak maps show delayed contrast agent bolus arrival in the right cortical region corresponding to the evolving DWI lesion. A perfusion deficit of the left precentral region appears to have resolved. (*Middle*) DWI performed within 40 minutes after onset of symptoms reveals a hyperacute ischemic lesion evolving in frontal and temporal right cortical regions involving the anterior and posterior operculum. In addition, the (3-day-old) acute lesion in the precentral region of the left cortex is well delineated. (*Bottom*) T$_2$-weighted images with no definite abnormality in the right hemisphere, but showing the small left precentral cortical region (arrow).

Diagnosis

Acute ischemic Foix–Chavany–Marie syndrome (FCMS).

General remarks

FCMS presents with anarthria and bilateral central facio-linguo-velo-pharyngeo-masticatory paralysis with "automatic voluntary dissociation." The most common cause of FCMS is cerebrovascular disease, while rarer etiologies also include central nervous system infection, developmental disorders, epilepsy, and neurodegenerative disorders. Even though this syndrome is also referred to as the "bilateral anterior operculum syndrome," patients with lesion sites other than both opercular cortices and even exceptional cases with unilateral lesions have been described.

Special remarks

This patient represents a typical case of FCMS as a consequence of two strokes in short succession in cortical areas that are likely to be functionally very closely related. The initial lesion affected only a relatively small area of the left pre-central cortex, while the second lesion was slightly more extensive involving parts of the right anterior and posterior operculum. Although severe functional deficits due to the simultaneous involvement of different cortical regions are only recognized in a few well-defined clinical syndromes in clinical practice such synergistic functional effects of focal lesions may be an important consideration in many stroke patients with multiple acute lesions or pre-existing lesions.

FIRST DESCRIPTION

Foix, C. & Chavany, J. A. Diplégies faciales d'origine corticale, avec quelques considér-ations sur les paralysies presudobulbaires et la localisation des centres corticaux de l'extrémité céphalique. *Ann. Méd.* 1926; **20**:480–498.

CURRENT REVIEW

Weller, M. Anterior opercular cortex lesions cause dissociated lower cranial nerve palsies and anarthria but no aphasia: Foix–Chavany–Marie syndrome and "automatic voluntary dissociation" revisited. *J. Neurol.* 1993; **240**:199–208.

SUGGESTED READING

Kobayashi, S., Kunimoto, M., & Takeda, K. A case of Foix–Chavany–Marie syndrome and crossed aphasia after right corona radiata infarction with history of left hemispheric infarction. *Rinsho Shinkeigaku* 1998; **38**:910–914.

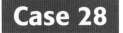

Severe headache and facial palsy

Clinical history

A 37-year-old woman with a 3-year history of hypertension presented with sudden onset, severe holocephalic headache. There was no impairment of consciousness or evidence of seizures. In the emergency department her blood pressure was 170/90 mm Hg.

Examination

The patient's Glasgow Coma Score was 15 and neurological examination showed nuchal rigidity as well as a peripheral facial palsy with slight hyperacusis and disturbance of taste.

Neurological scores

NIH 1; Barthel Index 90; GCS 15.

Special studies

Baseline cranial CT showed hyperdense blood signal in the prepontine and interpeduncular cisterns. On MRI, 2 days later no definite abnormality could be detected.

Follow-up

Follow-up CT 4 days later was normal. The patient recovered completely within 2 days.

Image findings

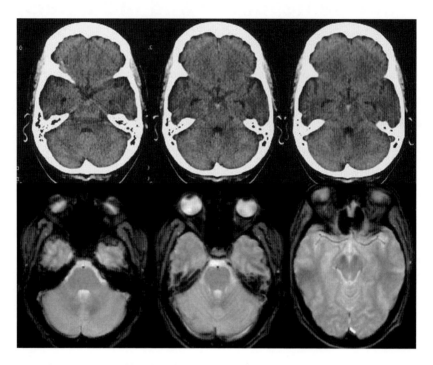

Figure 28.1 Hyperdense signal of blood in the prepontine and interpeduncular cisterns. MRI (2 days later) was normal – even susceptibility-weighted T_2^* sequences failed to identify at this timepoint the suspected hypodensity typically caused by deoxyhemoglobin.

Diagnosis

Perimesencephalic subarachnoid hemorrhage with transient affection of the facial nerve.

General remarks

In 15% to 20% of cases with perimesencephalic subarachnoid hemorrhage (pSAH) no causative source is found and conventional angiography is negative. Several studies have shown that patients with pSAH and a negative angiogram have a substantially better prognosis than patients with aneurysmal SAH. From the pattern of bleeding on CT or MRI, a particular subgroup of angiography negative patients with SAH could be identified with blood confined to the perimesencephalic cisterns. The risk of rebleeding is very low and the prognosis is excellent.

Special remarks

The absence of focal neurological deficits was considered as a typical clinical finding of pSAH. In a systematic literature review including 169 cases, there were only two cases with an impairment of the facial or the abducens nerves. However, it seems likely that, according to the distribution of the subarachnoid blood within the perimesencephalic cisterns, cranial nerves should be affected more frequently in pSAH. As presented in this case, only temporary impairment of cranial nerves might appear.

FIRST DESCRIPTION

van Gijn, J., van Dongen, K. J., Vermeulen, M., & Hijdra, A. Perimesencephalic hemorrhage: a nonaneurysmal and benign form of subarachnoid hemorrhage. *Neurology* 1985; **35**:493–497.

CURRENT REVIEW

Schwartz, T. H. & Solomon, R. A. Perimesencephalic nonaneurysmal subarachnoid hemorrhage: review of the literature. *Neurosurgery* 1996; **39**:433–440; discussion 440.

SUGGESTED READING

Arboix, A., Masson, J., Arribas, M. P., Oliveras, M., & Titus, F. Hemorragia perimesencefalica: una forma benigna de hemorragia subarachnoidea. *Neurologia* 1991; **6**:229–230.
Kitahara, T., Ohwada, T., Tokiwa, K. *et al.* Clinical studies in patients with perimesencephalic subarachnoid hemorrhage of unknown etiology. *No Shinkei Geka* 1993; **21**:903–908.
Rinkel, G. J., Wijdicks, E. F., Hasan, D. *et al.* Outcome in patients with subarachnoid haemorrhage and negative angiography according to pattern of haemorrhage on computed tomography. *Lancet* 1991; **338**:964–968.
Tubbs, R. S. & Oakes, W. J. Relationships of the cisternal segment of the trochlear nerve. *J. Neurosurg.* 1998; **89**:1015–1019.

Isolated difficulty, writing and grasping

Clinical history

A 75-year-old man noted weakness in his left hand making writing and grasping difficult for the last 8 hours. He described the symptom onset as sudden and reported no accompanying pain or abnormal sensations.

General history

Arterial hypertension, diabetes mellitus type 2.

Examination

On neurologic examination there was a pronounced ulnar distribution of left hand weakness (with involvement of the digits IV–V) with MRC grade 4 but full strength in all other digits. There was no additional clinical involvement of motor functions of the wrist or elbow or facial palsy. Shoulder strength and the ipsilateral lower extremity were not affected. A sensory deficit was not found.

Special studies

After unremarkable electromyographic studies of the ulnar nerve and an unrevealing CT scan, diffusion-weighted MRI demonstrated an acute ischemic lesion in the primary motor area of the hand in the precentral gyrus contralateral to the side of the weak hand. Additional vascular examinations including magnetic resonance angiography and ultrasound studies as well as further investigations for potential sources of embolus were negative.

Follow-up

In the following 7 days the neurological deficit resolved completely. He was treated with clopidogrel for secondary prophylaxis.

Image findings

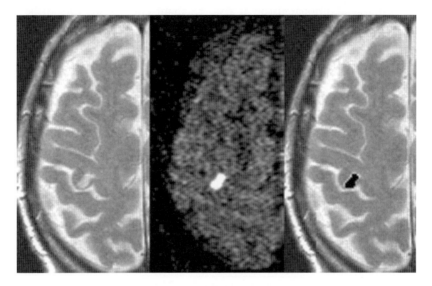

Figure 29.1 MRI was performed 12 hours after onset of left hand paresis (ulnar distribution). The acute lesion is identified on the diffusion-weighted image (b-factor = 1000 s/mm^2). The lesion is displayed as black pixels on the coregistered T$_2$-weighted image demonstrating its location in the medial aspect of the hand motor cortex.

Diagnosis

Acute ischemic distal arm paresis.

General remarks

Functional MRI studies have evaluated the representation of primary motor hand function and identified most frequently activation of the cortex in a specific region of the precentral gyrus. This area is localized to a knob-like segment of the precentral gyrus projecting to the middle genu of the central sulcus with a characteristic inverted omega or less often horizontal epsilon shape, termed the "hand knob."

Special remarks

Acute stroke with distal arm paresis can be a clinically challenging syndrome. The paucity of clinical signs may make it difficult to decide on its peripheral or central origin. Several studies have shown that acute ischemic distal arm paresis is usually caused by small cortical lesions due to embolic distal Rolandic artery obstruction without additional tissue at risk. Its main etiology appears to be cardiac and artery-to-artery embolism. The donor source is likely to produce very small particles such as white platelet-fibrin thrombi that block distal arterial branches. The offending vascular irregularities may be beyond detection by present imaging capabilities.

Partial hand knob lesions seem to indicate a somatotopic distribution of the hand motor cortex, which is not evident in larger lesions involving both lateral and medial zones of the hand knob.

SUGGESTED READING

Gass, A., Szabo, K., Behrens, S., Rossmanith, C., & Hennerici, M. A. Diffusion-weighted MRI study of acute ischemic distal arm paresis. *Neurology* 2001; **57**:1589–1594.

Jack, C. R., Jr., Thompson, R. M., Butts, R. K. *et al.* Sensory motor cortex: correlation of presurgical mapping with functional MR imaging and invasive cortical mapping. *Radiology* 1994; **190**:85–92.

Rao, S. M., Binder, J. R., Hammeke, T. A. *et al.* Somatotopic mapping of the human primary motor cortex with functional magnetic resonance imaging. *Neurology* 1995; **45**:919–924.

Tei, H. Monoparesis of the right hand following a localised infarct in the left "precentral knob." *Neuroradiology* 1999; **41**:269–270.

Yousry, T. A., Schmid, U. D., Alkadhi, H. *et al.* Localization of the motor hand area to a knob on the precentral gyrus. A new landmark. *Brain* 1997; **120**:141–157.

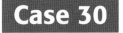

Young mother found comatose on the bathroom floor

Clinical history

A 41-year-old woman with no previous history of neurologic or cardiac illness was found comatose on the floor of her bathroom. She was last seen by her family 24 h earlier. According to her family, she smoked 20 cigarettes/day but was otherwise healthy.

Examination

Clinical examination of the comatose patient with a Glasgow Coma Score of 8 (eyes: 1, verbal: 2, motor function: 5) showed dilated unreactive pupils and Babinski signs on both sides. She showed decorticate posturing and a Cheyne–Stokes respiratory pattern. She had a heart rate of 90/min and a blood pressure of 110/75 mmHg.

Special studies

Cranial CT scan showed acute territorial infarctions in territories of three large brain supplying arteries (left MCA and PCA, and right MCA (Fig. 30.1a). Extra- and intracranial ultrasound showed bilateral middle cerebral artery and left internal carotid artery occlusions. In a transesophageal echocardiography performed on day 1, a mass lesion measuring 2.20 cm × 4.60 cm was seen in the left atrium prolapsing through the mitral valve (b).

Follow-up

On day 1, the patient showed slight spontaneous movement of her left leg and pain reaction on the left side of her body. On day 22, she was breathing by tracheostomy, showed decerebrate posturing and only an autonomic response to pain stimuli. She survived a further 9 months without any cerebral events before dying from pulmonary infection.

Image findings

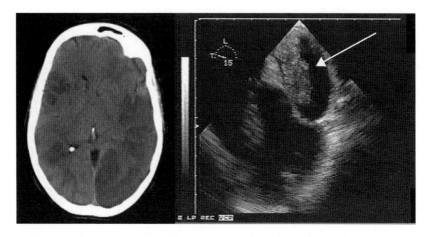

Figure 30.1 *Left image*: multiple brain infarction on cranial CT scan (MCA and PCA left and MCA right side). *Right image*: transesophageal echocardiography showing a floating mass lesion in the left atrium.

Diagnosis

Multiple brain embolism due to undiagnosed cardiac tumor.

General remarks

The incidence of cardiac tumors is low (0.05%), the most common being a myxoma. Approximately 75% of the patients with myxomas are women. The method of choice to detect a cardiac tumor is transesophageal echocardiography, and the most common and leading symptoms are arrhythmias and heart insufficiency. Some people predispose for cardiac emboli. Intracardiac tumors are responsible for less than 1% of all cerebral infarctions. Growth rates of 0.15 to 0.44 cm^2 per month may occur. The definitive treatment is surgical removal of myxomas with only a 0% to 3% operative mortality rate and a similar recurrence rate of 0% to 3%.

Stroke is the most common presentation of cardiac myxomas. The majority of reported infarcts are multiple, located in both hemispheres and more common in the left than in the right middle cerebral artery territory. In-hospital mortality was 27% in one series of myxoma patients. The factors that might be responsible for sudden unexpected symptoms are immunological metabolites involved in the development of cardiac emboli. Some discuss that the tumor has to reach a certain size when cardiac excitation is disturbed, to cause arrhythmias and emboli. Other data indicate that physical exercise can dislodge an embolus from a myxoma. The best time-point for surgery is not clear, as cardiopulmonary bypass and anticoagulation may exacerbate the neurological injury.

Special remarks

This patient is an example of how cardiac tumors can grow asymptomatically and stay undetected until the first symptoms arise and cause a life-threatening stroke. This underlines the necessity for early echocardiography in young patients with cryptogenic stroke. Because of the hereditary factor of atrial myxomas, it is recommended that echocardiography be performed in family members, particularly the young.

This patient is, however, remarkable because of two points. First, the myxoma became symptomatic by massive embolism to the brain without any prior cardiac abnormality or other warning signs and second because there were no further emboli despite conservative treatment with low-dose heparin only. Particularly, the second aspect is in contrast to other case descriptions that claim high rates of reembolization when full dose anticoagulation is performed.

FIRST DESCIPRTION

King, T. W. On simple vascular growths in the left auricle of the heart. *Lancet* 1845; 2:428–429.

CURRENT REVIEW

Reynen, K. 'Cardiac myxomas'. *N. Engl. J. Med.* 1995; **333**:1610–1617.

SUGGESTED READING

Bienfait, H. P. & Moll, L. C. Fatal cerebral embolism in a young patient with an occult left atrial myxoma. *Clin. Neurol. Neurosurg.* 2001; **103**:37–38.

Bulkley, B. H. & Hutchins, G. M. Atrial myxomas: a fifty year review. *Am. Heart J.* 1979; **97**:639–643.

Di Tullio, M. R. & Homma, S. Mechanisms of cardioembolic stroke. *Curr. Cardiol. Rep.* 2002; **4**:141–148.

Knepper, L. E., Biller, J., Adams, H. P., Jr., & Bruno, A. Neurologic manifestations of atrial myxoma. A 12-year experience and review. *Stroke* 1988; **19**:1435–1440.

Morton-Bours, E. C., Jacobs, M. B., & Albers, G. W. Clinical problem-solving. Eyes wide open. *N. Engl. J. Med.* 2000; **343**:50–55.

Pochis, W. T., Wingo, M. W., Cinquegrani, M. P., & Sagar, K. B. Echocardiographic demonstration of rapid growth of a left atrial myxoma. *Am. Heart J.* 1991; **122**: 1781–1784.

Shapiro, L. M. Cardiac tumours: diagnosis and management. *Heart* 2001; **85**:218–222.

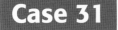

Case 31

Progressive mental decline and fever

Clinical history

A 66-year-old man with a 2-year course of progressive mental decline and a
2-week history of fever with episodes of severe confusion was admitted. While his
past medical history was unrevealing, his wife reported that one of his three
siblings, as well as his father, had died of "Alzheimer's disease."

Examination

On initial examination, the patient was oriented to self and time. He lacked
spontaneity and answered questions slowly and often after some delay. There
were no abnormalities of the cranial nerves, motor strength, reflexes, and sensory
functions.

Neurological scores

NIH 1; Barthel Index 70; GCS 15.

Special studies

Cranial MRI showed T2-hyperintense periventricular white matter lesions with
additional lacunar lesions in both cerebral hemispheres and especially in the
anterior temporal pole and the external capsule. DWI detected no acute ischemic
lesions. CSF analysis was normal. A urinary tract infection was treated with
antibiotics after which cognitive functions returned to the state, which the
patient's family considered as "normal." Neuropsychological testing including
the DemTect test identified signs of dementia (Demtect result 3/18; dementia is
considered with a score of 0–8 points).

Image findings

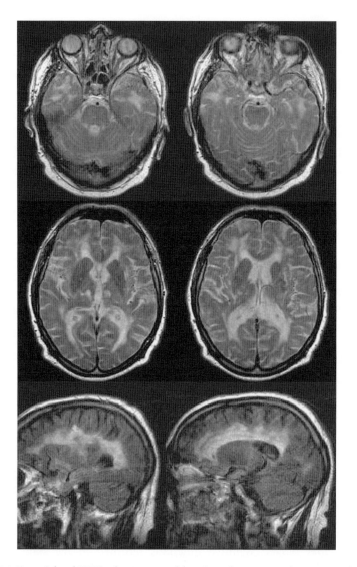

Figure 31.1 T$_2$-weighted MRI in the 66-year-old patient shows extensive symmetric hyperintense white-matter lesions involving the pons, the periventricular white matter, and especially the anterior temporal pole and the external capsule. Lacunar chronic ischemic lesions in the thalamus on both sides are seen.

Diagnosis

Cerebral autodominant arteriopathy with subcortical infarcts and leukoencephalopathy (CADASIL).

General remarks

CADASIL is a monogenic cause of ischemic small-vessel disease and stroke in middle-aged individuals. Clinical manifestations include TIAs and strokes (80%), cognitive deficits (50%), migraine with aura (40%), psychiatric disorders (30%), and epilepsy (10%). Mean age at onset is 46 years and MRI reveals a combination of small lacunar lesions and diffuse white matter abnormalities. Temporal pole T_2-hyperintensity is a radiologic marker of CADASIL as well as involvement of the external capsule and corpus callosum which are also characteristic findings that may help to distinguish the disease from SVE. The underlying vascular lesion is a unique non-amyloid angiopathy involving small arteries (100–4000 µm) and capillaries primarily in the brain. Diagnosis is made by skin biopsy. The disease is caused by mutations in the NOTCH3 gene, which codes for a large transmembrane receptor. CADASIL mutations involve highly conserved cysteine residues in epidermal-growth-factor-like repeat domains. Expression of NOTCH3 is restricted to vascular smooth-muscle cells. The mutations result in a selective accumulation of the extracellular domain of the receptor within blood vessels. New hereditary small vessel diseases distinct from NOTCH3 have recently been identified.

Special remarks

In our patient, the positive family history as well as the typical changes on MRI led us to consider CADASIL as a differential diagnosis. Diagnosis was then established with skin biopsy and genetic testing.

FIRST DESCRIPTION

Sourander, P. & Walinder, J. Hereditary multi-infarct dementia: morphological and clinical studies of a new disease. *Acta Neuropathol. (Berlin)* 1977; **39**:247–254.

SUGGESTED READING

Chabriat, H., Joutel, A., Vahedi, K. *et al.* [CADASIL (cerebral autosomal dominant arteriopathy with subcortical infarcts and leukoencephalopathy): clinical features and neuroimaging]. *Bull. Acad. Natl Med.* 2000; **184**:1523–1531; discussion 1531–1533.

Joutel, A., Favrole, P., Labauge, P. *et al.* Skin biopsy immunostaining with a Notch3 monoclonal antibody for CADASIL diagnosis. *Lancet* 2001; **358**:2049–2051.

Joutel, A., Francois, A., Chabriat, H. *et al.* [CADASIL: genetics and physiopathology]. *Bull. Acad. Natl Med.* 2000; **184**:1535–1542; discussion 1542–1544.

O'Sullivan, M., Jarosz, J. M., Martin, R. J., Deasy, N., Powell, J. F., & Markus, H. S. MRI hyperintensities of the temporal lobe and external capsule in patients with CADASIL. *Neurology* 2001; **56**:628–634.

Verreault, S., Joutel, A., Riant, F. *et al.* A novel hereditary small vessel disease of the brain. *Ann. Neurol.* 2006; **59**:353–357.

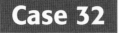

Aphasia after laparoscopic cholecystectomy

Clinical history

A 57-year-old man underwent a laparoscopic cholecystectomy for acute chole-cystitis caused by cholecystolithiasis. The laparoscopic procedure, associated with an increased intraperitoneal pressure due to gas insufflation, was surgically uncomplicated. Three hours after the operation, during the recovery phase, right sided sensorimotor hemiparesis and global aphasia were noted.

General history

Malignant melanoma at the right thigh with regional lymph node metastases 5 years ago, reflux esophagitis.

Examination

On neurological examination, the patient was alert, but had no verbal comprehension or response and only slight proximal motor function of the right arm and leg.

Neurological scores on admission

NIH 18; Barthel Index 5; GCS 9.

Special studies

Immediately performed CCT showed early signs of infarction, caused by a proximal occlusion of the left MCA with a hyperdense MCA sign. Stroke was confirmed by subsequent MRI including MR angiography with spontaneous recanalization of the left MCA. Duplex ultrasound showed an occlusion of the left ICA. Transesophageal echocardiography showed a large PFO III° with an atrial septal aneurysm and right-to-left shunting during Valsalva maneuver following contrast injection. Along with an elevated titer of D-dimer, a clinically asymptomatic thrombosis of the medial gastrocnemius veins as the cause of the embolism was identified on duplex ultrasound. Further investigation excluded other causes for cardiac embolism as well as a carotid dissection or significant carotid atherosclerosis. Clotting studies revealed no signs of a hypercoagulable disorder.

Follow-up

The patient received treatment with low-molecular-weight heparin followed by anticoagulation with phenprocoumon (INR 2.0 to 2.5). During the hospital stay the headache improved completely, but the patient developed transient symptoms of dizziness, diplopia, and transient sensory loss in the ulnar area of the right hand. MRI follow-up did not show any signs of hemorrhage or ischemia. In the 3-month follow-up the patient had fully recovered and the MRI scan displayed completely reopened cerebral venous system. The anticoagulative treatment was replaced by a platelet function inhibitor (Clopidogrel 75 mg/d).

Image findings

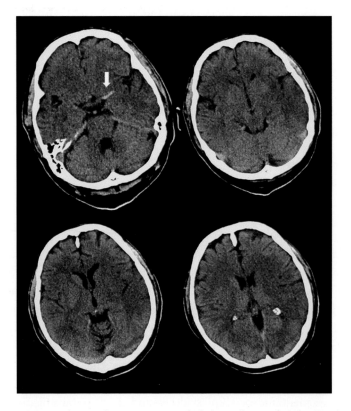

Figure 32.1 CT-Scan 4 hours after surgery revealed signs of an early infarction in the territory of the left middle cerebral artery with a hyperdense MCA-sign (arrow), cortical effacement, edema in the lenticular nucleus (lower left image) and demarcation in the temporal lobe (upper right image).

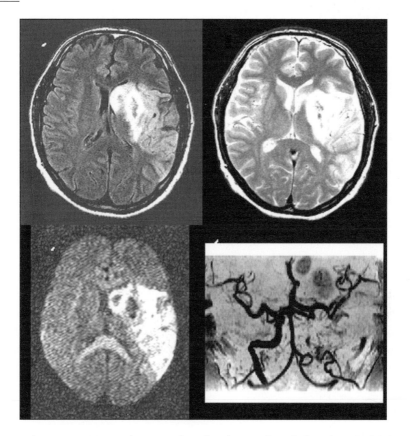

Figure 32.2 Subsequent MRI on day 7 confirmed a large subcortical and cortical infarction in the territory of the left middle cerebral artery (axial images: upper left FLAIR, upper right T$_2$-weighted, lower left diffusion-weighted), MR-angiography revealed an occlusion of the left ICA and an early recanalization of the left MCA (lower right).

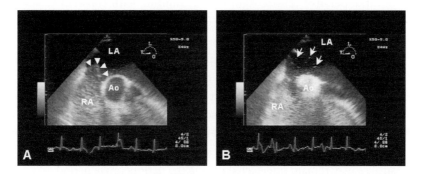

Figure 32.3 Transesophageal echocardiography showed PFO with aneurysm of atrial septum and right-to-left shunting during Valsalva maneuver following contrast injection (A) contrast bubbles in right atrium, aneurysm of atrial septum (arrowheads); (B) detection of bubbles (arrows) in left atrium within three heart cycles. Ao, aorta; LA, left atrium, RA, right atrium.

Diagnosis

Ischemic stroke in the distribution of the left MCA due to paradoxical embolism after laparoscopic procedure in a patient with PFO.

General remarks

Paradoxical embolism of thrombi arising in the venous system and passing via a transient right-to-left shunt at the level of the atria is the postulated main stroke mechanism in patients with PFO. However, there are only few reported cases of a proven thrombus traversing a PFO. Alternatively, thrombembolism from atrial septal aneurysms or secondary cardiac arrhythmias serving as stroke etiologies apart from paradoxical embolism are discussed.

Recently, a series of four patients was reported with PFO who had strokes develop during sexual intercourse. Paradoxical embolization as a result of the elevated intrathoracic pressure during sexual activity as the probable stroke mechanism was proposed, although the source of embolism was not identified in any of these patients. Further case reports strengthen the association of stroke and paradoxical embolism to scuba diving and laparoscopic procedures in patients with large PFO.

Special remarks

As a result of the pneumoperitoneum during laparoscopic procedures central venous pressure exceeds pulmonary wedge pressure, leading to temporary reversal of intracardiac pressure gradients between the atria. In consequence, the risk of intraoperative cardiac right-to-left shunting with consecutive systemic embolisation is increased, because a PFO, although normally closed, may open during this reversal of pressure gradients.

Potential sources of paradoxical embolism such as deep vein thrombosis are detected only in a minority of cases (4%–10%), despite extensive diagnostic work-up. According to the high prevalence of a PFO (approximately 27%) and the increasing frequency of laparoscopic procedures, a higher incidence of stroke as the few cases described in literature might be expected. Presumably, the preoperative incidence of deep vein thrombosis as the source of embolism is very low, and minor strokes may remain undetected during the perioperative period.

CURRENT REVIEW

Horton, S. C. & Bunch, T. J. Patent foramen ovale and stroke. *Mayo Clin. Proc.* 2004; **79**:79–88.

SUGGESTED READING

Becker, K., Skalabrin, E., Hallam, D., & Gill, E. Ischemic stroke during sexual intercourse. *Arch. Neurol.* 2004; **61**:1114–1116.

Hirvonen, E. A., Nuutinen, L. S., & Kauko, M. Hemodynamic changes due to Trendelen-burg positioning and pneumoperitoneum during laparoscopic hysterectomy. *Acta Anaesthesiol. Scand.* 1995; **39**:949–955.

Knauth, M., Ries, S., Pohimann, S. *et al.* Cohort study of multiple brain lesions in sport divers: role of a patent foramen ovale. *Br. Med. J.* 1997; **314**:701–705.

Lethen, H., Flachskampf, F. A., Schneider, R. *et al.* Frequency of deep vein thrombosis in patients with a patent foramen ovale and ischemic stroke or transient ischemic attack. *Am. J. Cardiol.* 1997; **80**:1066–1069.

Mandorla, S., Fronticelli, M., & Taliani, M. R. Pulmonary embolism and cerebral stroke from paradoxical embolism in a young woman. *G. Ital. Cardiol.* 1997; **27**:588–592.

Messé, S. R., Silverman, I. E., Kizer, J. R. *et al.* Practice parameter: recurrent stroke with patent foramen ovale and atrial septal aneurysm: Report of the Quality Standards Subcommittee of the American Academy of Neurology. *Neurology* 2004; **62**:1042–1050.

Salonen, M., Mäkinen, J., Saraste, M., & Parkkola, R. Is laparoscopic hysterectomy bad for the brain? *Gyn. Endoscop.* 1999; **8**:161–164.

Risks of carotid surgery in longstanding asymptomatic disease

Clinical history

A 61-year-old asymptomatic woman with known occlusion of the right common carotid artery was admitted when after years of regular follow-up ultrasound examinations a previously stable left ICA stenosis progressed from 60% to 90%. Apart from hypertension, there were no cardiovascular risk factors. On admission, she had no focal neurological deficit. The decision for surgery on the left ICA was made based on rapidly progressing severe extracranial vessel disease.

Examination

Immediately after surgery, the patient had an episode of slight transient hemiparesis on the right side of her body. On the second day after surgery, persisting left-sided brachiofacial hemiparesis occurred. On diffusion-weighted MRI a small embolic lesion of the hemisphere ipsilateral to the endarterectomy and a larger contralateral subcortical ischemic lesion were detected. On the fourth postoperative day, severe clinical deterioration was observed with alteration of consciousness, anisocoria, conjugate deviation of the eyes to the right and severe left hemiplegia.

Neurological scores on day 4
NIH 18; Barthel Index 0; GCS 11.

Special studies

MRI showed extensive subcortical infarction in the region of the right anterior and middle cerebral artery with a perfusion deficit of the complete right hemisphere. MRA revealed continuous flow signal in all intracranial vessels of the right hemisphere; however, with reduced intensity in comparison to the preoperative MRI. Repeat Doppler follow-up studies failed to show signs of re-stenosis of the left ICA and confirmed the persistence of the preoperative collateralization pattern of the right hemisphere with retrograde flow in the right ACA and, to a lesser extent, the participation of the posterior circulation via the right posterior communicating artery.

Follow-up

Follow-up MRI 2 months, 1 year and 2 years after surgery displayed an unusual distribution of infarction with thinning of areas of the cortex and a high intensity signal along the gyri. In contrast to the typical course of territorial infarction after recanalization of an occluded distal vessel, the images suggested extensive but incomplete cortical and subcortical tissue destruction in the hypoperfused regions. Accordingly, color-coded diffusion tensor images revealed extensive tissue destruction in the right MCA and ACA territory.

Image findings

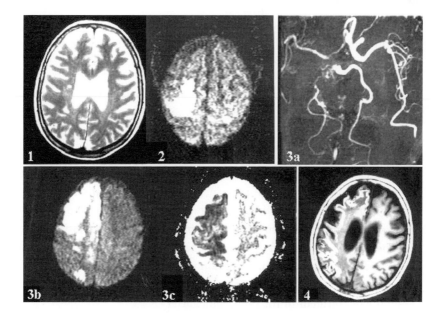

Figure 33.1 On preoperative T_2-weighted images slight cortical widening and two lesions in the deep white matter are seen (1). Emergency MRI on the second postoperative day revealed early signs of bilateral acute cortical ischemic lesions on the diffusion-weighted image within the MCA territory (2). On day 4 MRA (3a) showed patent flow signal in the proximal MCA but some distal flow signal loss and a reduction of flow signal in the right ACA and MCA. Early signs of extensive anterior and middle cerebral artery territory infarction of the right hemisphere are seen as hyperintense cortical and subcortical lesions on the diffusion weighted image and map of the apparent diffusion coefficient (3b, c). Follow-up MRI showed signs of extensive cortical ischemic damage as a hyperintense band on T_1-weighted images (4).

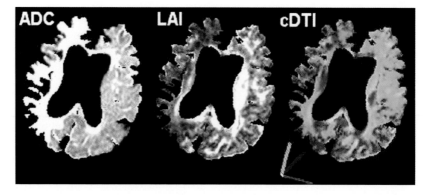

Figure 33.2 DWI including ADC, lattice anisotropy index maps and color-coded diffusion tensor images 2 years after stroke show extensive tissue destruction in the right MCA and ACA territory despite relative tissue preservation in the T_1-weighted image (see Fig. 33.1(4)).

Diagnosis

MR features of incomplete ischemia in progressive peri- and postoperative stroke contralateral to carotid endarterectomy in an asymptomatic woman with long-standing bilateral severe carotid disease.

General remarks

In several surgical and neurological reviews, perioperative stroke *contralateral* to the side of carotid endarterectomy has been reported in patients with an occluded contralateral carotid artery. Although some of the cases were attributed to perioperative systemic hypotension, no further investigation has been performed in order to define the underlying pathogenic mechanism or to analyze the pattern of infarction. It has been shown that in the occlusion-stenosis group, the hemisphere over the occluded artery is hemodynamically impaired. Our patient's preoperative hemodynamic situation was characterized by stable collateralization both via the anterior and the posterior communicating arteries and, in addition, by the recruitment of the ophthalmic artery.

Special remarks

Since in our case no episode of systemic hypotension was documented perioperatively, the mechanism of postoperative infarctions in the right hemisphere is not obvious. From the fact that an embolic lesion was present on the operated side, a cross-embolization can be hypothesized as the cause of subcortical MCA infarction, although thousands of TCD monitoring studies never demonstrated such a mechanism to be relevant. Moreover, an embolic mechanism alone would not explain the persistent severe hypoperfusion of the right hemisphere, which was especially accentuated in the hemodynamic risk zones between the MCA and ACA territories. This topographical distribution of ischemic injury seen in MRI leads us to favor a combination of pathomechanisms assuming a transient occlusion of the anterior collateralization pathway (possibly of embolic origin) and a decreased blood supply via the posterior communicating artery due to redistribution of blood flow following carotid endarterectomy. Evidence for such a blood flow reduction in the vertebro-basilar system after carotid endarterectomy has been provided by Blankenstejn *et al.* The theory of multiple underlying mechanisms is supported by follow-up MRI results, collected up to 2 years after surgery, that showed thinning of the cortical layers and a high intensity signal along the gyri with persistent hypoperfusion in large parts of the hemisphere. The area of hypoperfusion substantially exceeded the zones of complete infarction as reflected by chronic lesions. MRI follow-up findings in our case were in line with such a pathomechanism, suggesting that either embolic ischemia with fast spontaneous clot resolution and/or hypoperfusion due to decompensation of critical hypoperfusion after CEA might have happened. The theory of selective vulnerability and the selective neuronal loss termed "incomplete infarction" has been shown in experimental models after transient occlusion of an intracranial artery. Although the concept of incomplete stroke is rarely applied to human stroke, our report suggests – on the basis of morphological and functional features – the involvement of such a mechanism.

FIRST DESCRIPTION

Scholz, W. Die nicht zur Erweichung führenden unvollständigen Gewebsnecrosen (Elektive Parenchymnekrose). In Lubarsch, O., Rössle, R. & Henke, F., eds. *Handbuch der speziellen pathologischen Anatomie und Histologie*, XIII: Band, Nervensystem, 1:Teil, Bandteil B. Berlin/Göttingen/Heidelberg: Springer Verlag, 1957; 1284–1325.

SUGGESTED READING

Balotta, E., Da Giau, G., & Guerra, M. Carotid endarterectomy and contralateral internal carotid artery occlusion: Perioperative risks and long-term-stroke and survival rates. *Surgery* 1998; **23**:234–240.

Baron, J. C. Stroke research in the modern era: images versus dogmas. *Cerebrovasc. Dis.* 2005; **20**:154–163.

Blankensteijn, J. D., van der Grond, J., Mali, W. P., & Eikelboom, B. C. Flow volume changes in the major cerebral arteries before and after carotid endarterectomy: an MR angiography study. *Eur. J. Vasc. Endovasc. Surg.* 1997; **14**:446–450.

Garcia, J. H., Lassen, N. A., Weiller, C., Sperling, B., & Nakagawara, J. Ischemic stroke and incomplete infarction. *Stroke* 1996; **27**:761–765.

Kluytmans, M., van der Grond, J., Eikelboom, B. C., & Viergever, M. A. Long-term hemodynamic effects of carotid endarterectomy. *Stroke* 1998; **29**:1567–1572.

Moustafa, R. R. & Baron, J. C. Imaging the penumbra in acute stroke. *Curr. Atheroscler. Rep.* 2006; **8**:281–289.

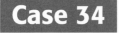

Recurrent weakness after major car accident

Clinical history

A 19-year-old, fully conscious man was admitted with an acute left hemiparesis. His history included a similar episode 1 year earlier with complete recovery, and a major car accident as a front seat passenger 3 years previously. At that time, he had injured his abdomen and legs; however, no chest or neck trauma was reported.

Examination

Examination showed sensorimotor brachio-facial hemiparesis on the left side and discrete swelling in the right supraclavicular fossa.

Neurological scores

NIH 8; Barthel Index 60; GCS 15.

Special studies

MRI showed old vascular lesions in the centrum semiovale and basal ganglia in the right cerebral hemisphere. Diffusion-weighted imaging showed an acute infarct in the right basal ganglia, posterolateral to the old lesion. No apparent source of embolism was revealed by extensive cardiovascular examination. Extra-cranial color Doppler/duplex-sonography demonstrated a pseudoaneurysm of the lateral wall of the right carotid bulb containing echolucent thrombus and an ectatic subclavian artery. Conventional angiography confirmed the sonographic findings.

Follow-up

A surgical removal of the pseudoaneurysm was performed, and then endarterectomy completed by a saphenous graft. After 3 weeks, the patient was discharged to a rehabilitation center. After 1 year, he showed stable slight functional impairment mRS 1 (NIH 2).

Image findings

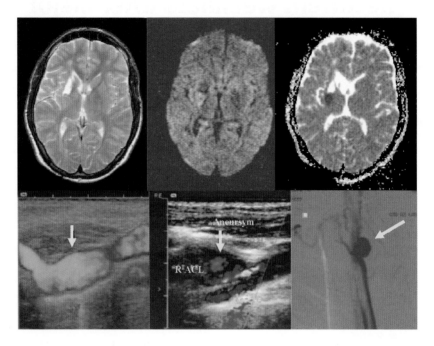

Figure 34.1 T_2-weighted image shows old ischemic lesions in the basal ganglia (upper left) while DWI (upper middle) and maps of the ADC (upper right) reveal an acute lesion in the basal ganglia posterolateral to the chronic stroke. Color Doppler sonography shows an aneurysm of the right carotid bifurcation and ecstasia of the subclavian artery (lower left and middle) confirmed by conventional angiography (lower right).

Diagnosis

Recurrent embolism from traumatic aneurysm of the ICA and right subclavian artery.

General remarks

Dissection of the extracranial portion of the carotid artery presents most commonly with symptoms of cerebral ischemia, either as fixed (50% of cases) or transient neurologic deficits (30% of cases), characteristically in association with pain in the side of the neck, face, or head ipsilateral to the carotid artery affected. Isolated pain in these locations is seen in approximately 15% of patients. The pain and headache may be mild or severe, sometimes resembling that of migraine, (including migrainous aura), but frequently it is dull and nonthrobbing. Several aspects of the clinical history and physical examination should prompt the clinician to consider the diagnosis of additional traumatic aneurysm particularly the association of an acute focal neurological deficit with pain in the neck, face, or head, pulsatile tinnitus, a new bruit, or Horner syndrome ipsilateral to the carotid artery affected. In addition, carotid artery dissection should be in the differential diagnosis of isolated cranial nerve pareses, particularly the lower cranial nerves. Carotid dissection should be part of the differential diagnosis of patients who present with isolated Horner syndrome or acute and severe headaches.

Special remarks

First reported in 1872 by Verneuil, according to scarce data traumatic injury of the common or internal carotid artery occurs in 1–10 in 1000 blunt injuries. Delayed ischemic events of the brain have been reported up to 15 years after trauma. Traumatic dissection of the cervical carotid artery reflects the fact that the pharyngeal (extracranial) portion of the vessel, like sections of the vertebral artery and aorta, is mobile; other vessels of similar size, such as the coronary and renal arteries, are fixed in place and less likely to dissect due to trauma. The prepetrous segment of the internal carotid, from its origin at the carotid bulb to entry into the petrous portion of the temporal bone, is commonly implicated. The internal carotid artery is compressed against the transverse processes of upper cervical vertebra and a hematoma forms on the posterior internal carotid artery wall. As in our case, seat belt pressure can cause vascular lesions and can consequence aneurysm and stroke. Surgical resection and endovascular stenting are competing methods for vessel repair.

FIRST DESCRIPTION

Verneuil, M. Confusions multiples; dé lire violent; hémiplegie à droite, Signes de compression cérébrale. *Bull. Acad. Med. (Paris)* 1872; **36**:46–56.

SUGGESTED READING

Benito, M. C., Garcia, F., Fernandez-Quero, L. *et al.* Lesion of the internal carotid artery caused by a car safety belt. *J. Trauma* 1990; **30**:116–117.

Fusonie, G. E., Edwards, J. D., & Reed, A. B. Covered stent exclusion of blunt traumatic carotid artery pseudoaneurysm: case report and review of the literature. *Ann. Vasc. Surg.* 2004; **18**:376–379.

McConnell, E. J. & Macbeth, G. A. Common carotid artery and tracheal injury from shoulder strap seat belt. *J. Trauma* 1997; **43**:150–152.

Mayberry, J. C., Brown, C. V., Mullins, R. J., & Velmahos, G. C. Blunt carotid artery injury: the futility of aggressive screening and diagnosis. *Arch. Surg.* 2004; **139**:609–612.

Pozzati, E., Giuliani, G., Poppi, M., & Faenza A. Blunt traumatic carotid dissection with delayed symptoms. *Stroke* 1989; **20**:412–416.

Prall, J. A., Brega, K. E., Coldwell, D. M., & Breeze, R. E. Incidence of unsuspected blunt carotid artery injury. *Neurosurgery* 1998; **42**:495–498.

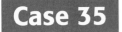

Stroke at awakening

Clinical history

A 54-year-old right-handed woman suddenly developed left-sided limb weakness. She had noticed her symptoms when she awoke at 7o'clock. Since she had gone to the bathroom 1.5 hours earlier without any deficit, the time window of stroke onset upon arrival in the emergency department at 9.30 was estimated to be between 2.5 and 4 hours. Past medical history was negative except for an occlusion of the central retinal artery 3 years ago, but there was no history of previous stroke or myocardial infarction. The patient is a smoker with approximately 30-pack–years.

Examination

Neurological deficit consisted in a mild dysarthria, severe left-sided limb weakness, left limb hypesthesia and mild facial palsy with positive Babinski sign on the left.

Neurological scores

NIH 13, Barthel-Index 35, GCS 14.

Special studies

On admission, ECG and routine laboratory tests were normal. Due to the undefined time window, the patient underwent immediate stroke MRI instead of a CT scan. Diffusion-weighted MRI (DWI) demonstrated an early ischemic lesion in the right insular cortex, parietal subcortical region and lateral basal ganglia, while perfusion-weighted MRI (PWI) showed a delayed contrast bolus arrival in the complete right MCA territory indicating this region to be at risk of infarction ("DWI/PWI-mismatch"). Correspondingly, MRA showed persistent occlusion of the M1 segment of the right MCA/ICA (a). There were no signs of intracranial hemorrhage on T_2^*- or FLAIR images. Supported by the finding of "tissue at risk" and persistent vascular occlusion, the patient was transferred to the stroke unit and underwent intravenous thrombolysis with r-tPA, despite the time window being possibly more than 3 hours.

Follow-up

Already during thrombolysis, the patient's symptoms improved to an NIHSS of 7. On follow-up, MRI performed 12 hours after thrombolysis, PWI deficits resolved and most of the previously hypoperfused tissue was salvaged. MRA showed recanalization of the right MCA (b). One week later, the patient was transferred to a rehabilitation center with only slight residual facial and upper extremity paresis (NIHSS 3).

Image findings

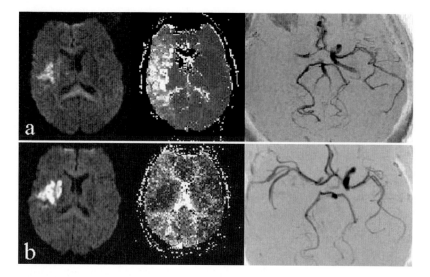

Figure 35.1 MRI-guided therapy decision in a 54-year-old woman with estimated onset of symptoms 2.5 to 4 hours earlier. (a) Demonstrates DWI/PWI mismatch with the right MCA territory at risk of infarction, while MRA shows M1 occlusion. On follow-up MRI 12 hours after thrombolysis (b), PWI deficits have resolved and most of hypoperfused tissue has been salvaged. MRA demonstrates recanalization of the right MCA.

Diagnosis

Acute embolic infarction in the right MCA territory with unknown onset of stroke symptoms. MRI-guided thrombolysis after a presumed time window of 2.5 to 4 hours.

General remarks

Even though thrombolysis has not yet been shown to be effective beyond the 3-hour time window, meta-analyses suggest a positive effect when given 3–6 hours after stroke onset. If extending the time window would prove to be successful, it would enable a more widespread use of thrombolytics in acute stroke therapy. Until then, one approach is the so-called MRI-guided patient selection, using perfusion and diffusion-weighted MRI to identify patients with a PWI/DWI-mismatch, as patients who might potentially benefit from recanalizing therapy.

Special remarks

This is an example of a patient who received i.v. thrombolysis after a presumed time window of 3–5 hours and after MRI identified her as someone at potential benefit to treatment. In this situation, MRI may offer a method that can help in the estimation of irreversibly injured and potentially salvageable tissue when 3 hours have already passed since the onset. In a recent MRI guided study (DIAS) of patients selected according to a PWI > DWI mismatch, those patients treated with thrombolysis in a 3–9 h time window had comparable outcomes to the 3 h NINDS trial results. To extend the time window beyond 3 hrs even without MR imaging, ECASS III (European Cooperative Acute Stroke Study), a multicenter, randomized, double-blind, placebo-controlled trial in 110 hospitals in 15 European countries is ongoing and evaluates the efficacy and safety of rt-PA between 3 and 4.5 hours after stroke onset.

SUGGESTED READING

Hacke, W., Albers, G., Al-Rawi, Y. *et al.* DIAS Study Group. The Desmoteplase in Acute Ischemic Stroke Trial (DIAS): a phase II MRI-based 9-hour window acute stroke thrombolysis trial with intravenous desmoteplase. *Stroke* 2005; 36:66–73.

Ingall, T. J., O'Fallon, W. M., Asplund, K. *et al.* Findings from the reanalysis of the NINDS tissue plasminogen activator for acute ischemic stroke treatment trial. *Stroke* 2004; 35:2418–2424.

Kohrmann, M., Juttler, E., Fiebach, J. B. *et al.* MRI versus CT-based thrombolysis treatment within and beyond the 3 h time window after stroke onset: a cohort study. *Lancet Neurol.* 2006; 5:661–667.

Röther, J., Schellinger, P. D., Gass, A. *et al.* Kompetenznetzwerk Schlaganfall Study Group. Effect of intravenous thrombolysis on MRI parameters and functional outcome in acute stroke <6 hours. *Stroke* 2002; 33:2438–2445.

Case 36

Cognitive impairment and seizures

Clinical history

A 51-year-old right-handed man had a first-ever generalized epileptic seizure preceded by a rapidly developing cognitive decline, confusion, and sensory aphasia. His past medical history was negative except for persistent headaches of moderate intensity during the last 2 weeks and a history of controlled hypertension and hypercholesterolemia. In particular, there was no evidence for any previous cerebrovascular event; his family history was also negative.

Examination

On admission, he was confused, not oriented to place and time, and he was not able to name his wife. A complex neuropsychological syndrome was present with sensory aphasia, dyscalculia, dyslexia, motor dyspraxia, visual agnosia and right visual hemineglect. The clinical examination revealed no further abnormality of motor, sensory or coordination function.

Neurological scores

NIH 10; Barthel Index 50; GCS 13.

Special studies

MRI was performed showing diffuse hyperintensity on T_2-weighted sequences and FLAIR images, extensively involving subcortical areas of the left temporal, parietal and occipital lobes as well as of the right parietal lobe, including the subcortical U-fibers, with slight mass effect and effacement of the sulci (a). Abnormal enhancement was absent after gadolinium injection. A residuum of lobar hemorrhage was detected on T_2^*-gradient-echo weighted sequences in the right parieto-occipital region. Furthermore, there were multiple, widespread punctuate areas of low intensity in both hemispheres suggestive of chronic microbleedings, mainly in cortical and corticosubcortical location. Analysis of CSF showed no abnormalities except for an elevated total protein level of 1030 mg/l. Electroencephalography revealed a continuous left parieto-occipital rhythmic delta focus mixed with sharp waves compatible with non-convulsive complex partial status epilepticus.

Thirteen days after admission, cortical and leptomeningeal biopsies were taken from the left parieto-occipital lesion. Eosinophilic wall thickening of cortical arterioles and leptomeningeal arteries was present, the eosinophilic material stained with Congo red showed apple green birefringence when observed with the polarizing microscope, which is diagnostic of amyloid angiopathy.

Follow-up

During the 3-week hospital stay, the patient had some gradual recovery. He received intravenous aciclovir until the exclusion of herpes simplex encephalitis; under anticonvulsive treatment with valproate both cognitive impairment and electroencephalography (EEG) findings improved. The patient was discharged with only minimal residual aphasia and memory disturbances. Four months later, he was rehospitalized due to recurrent focal seizures. During these 4 months, he had recovered progressively and had almost achieved his cognitive baseline. MRI now revealed significant regression of the diffuse T_2-hyperintense abnormalities (b).

Image findings

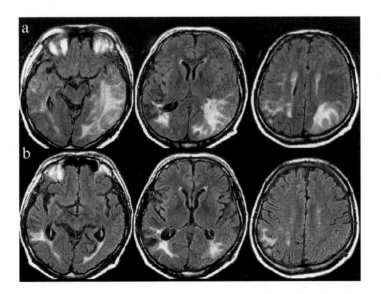

Figure 36.1 (a) MRI performed 6 hours after admission. FLAIR images show diffuse hyperintensity involving subcortical areas of the left temporal, parietal and occipital lobes as well as of the right parietal lobe involving the subcortical U-fibers.

Diagnosis

CAA presenting as reversible leukoencephalopathy without acute intracerebral hemorrhage.

General remarks

CAA is characterized by the deposition of homogeneous eosinophilic material in the media and adventitia of arterioles and small arteries of the cortex and leptomeninges. It commonly occurs in the aging brain and is found in approximately 30% of elderly asymptomatic patients. CAA is usually asymptomatic, until spontaneous intracerebral hemorrhages occur as the most common first clinical presentation. CAA-related hemorrhages mostly occur in corticosubcortical (or lobar) brain regions. CAA-related hemorrhages are often multiple and recurrent. Other clinical features include dementia, seizures, cerebral ischemia, and leukoencephalopathy. Gray *et al.* first described severe white matter changes in 8 of 12 brains of patients with diffuse hemorrhagic CAA. These white matter changes were distributed similar to those observed in SVE which most predominantly affects periventricular areas and spares U-fibers, corpus callosum, and internal capsules. A pathomechanism of chronic hypoperfusion in the deep white matter due to amyloid-related small vessel disease of long perforating arterioles was posited to be the cause of leukoencephalopathy.

Special remarks

Caulo *et al.* first described a patient with a dynamic course of CAA-related leukoencephalopathy located in both subcortical and lobar structures of both hemispheres, with absence of intracranial hemorrhage and showing both signs of progression as well as regressive changes in a follow-up MRI after 1 year. Recently, other patients with dynamic and/or regressive courses in CAA-related leukoencephalopathy have been reported; common clinical manifestations were cognitive decline, personality changes, aphasia, seizures, gait disturbances and headaches. Similar to our patient, all descriptions of CAA-related leukoencephalopathy with dynamic clinical course and neuroimaging signs of disease regression showed markedly different characteristics to the white matter changes (similar to SVE)

Caption for Fig. 36.1 (*cont.*)
Mild signs of mass effect and effacement of the sulci are present. (b) Follow-up MRI after 4 months. FLAIR images now demonstrates a clear regression of the diffuse subcortical hyperintensities with only mild residual changes in both parieto-occipital regions.

that were described in the neuropathological study of Gray *et al.* This implicates the existence of two subcategories of white matter changes related to CAA. First, the "periventricular" and symmetrical form which spares the U-fibers may slowly progress, has a high incidence but is non-specific, may correlate with the severity of CAA, and be associated with a higher risk of spontaneous hemorrhage. Second, the less common, "lobar" form of leukoencephalopathy involves the U-fibers, may present with or without intracerebral hemorrhage, but does not appear to correlate with the severity of CAA and may be reversible under certain conditions. So far, no systematic data are available on the follow-up of both clinical conditions in a prospective series of patients. A pathomechanism of perivascular inflammation evoked by vascular amyloid deposition and subsequent vascular dysfunction has recently been suggested to be responsible for the reversible leukoencephalopathy syndrome.

SUGGESTED READING

Caulo, M., Tampieri, D., Brassard, R., Christine, G. M., & Melanson, D. Cerebral amyloid angiopathy presenting as nonhemorrhagic diffuse encephalopathy: neuropathologic and neuroradiologic manifestations in one case. *Am. J. Neuroradiol.* 2001; **22**:1072–1076.

Eng, J. A., Frosch, M. P., Choi, K., Rebeck, G. W., & Greenberg, S. M. Clinical manifestations of cerebral amyloid angiopathy-related inflammation. *Ann. Neurol.* 2004; **55**: 250–256.

Gray, F., Dubas, F., Roullet, E., & Escourolle, R. Leukoencephalopathy in diffuse hemorrhagic cerebral amyloid angiopathy. *Ann. Neurol.* 1985; **18**:54–59.

Greenberg, S. M., Vonsattel, J. P., Stakes, J. W., Gruber, M., & Finklestein, S. P. The clinical spectrum of cerebral amyloid angiopathy: presentations without lobar hemorrhage. *Neurology* 1993; **43**:2073–2079.

Oh, U., Gupta, R., Krakauer, J. W., Khandji, A. G., Chin, S. S., & Elkind, M. S. Reversible leukoencephalopathy associated with cerebral amyloid angiopathy. *Neurology* 2004; **62**:494–497.

Vinters, H. V. Cerebral amyloid angiopathy. A critical review. *Stroke* 1987; **18**:311–324.

Yamada, M. Cerebral amyloid angiopathy: an overview. *Neuropathology* 2000; **20**:8–22.

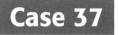

Progressive headache, tinnitus, and nausea

Clinical history

A 53-year-old man with a 6-hour history of progressively worsening headache associated with tinnitus, nausea, and vomiting was found unresponsive at home by his father. Paramedics reported a hemiparesis on the right, dysarthria and a previously unknown cardiac arrhythmia on ECG.

He had a 2-year history of hypertension, but was not known to have other medical conditions.

Examination

Neurologic examination on admission showed an obtunded patient who opened his eyes to painful stimulation, but did not follow instructions or communicate. The eyes were conjugately deviated to the right and he had a slight sensorimotor palsy on the right side predominantly involving the face and upper limb.

Neurological scores

NIH 11; Barthel Index 0; GCS 9.

Special studies

After a non-revealing CT scan, MRI was performed showing acute cerebellar infarcts in the left PICA and SCA territory as well as an acute subcortical stroke in the left MCA territory. Atrial fibrillation on ECG confirmed the suspected cardiac source of embolism. Ultrasound was normal except for a hypoplastic left vertebral artery. During the course of 48 hours the patient became comatose with a GCS of 5, had anisocoria R > L and skew deviation. CT scan now showed a well-demarcated cerebellar infarct with brain stem compression by mass effect and occlusion of the cerebral aqueduct. A suboccipital craniectomy with evacuation of infarcted tissue and temporizing ventriculostomy were performed.

Follow-up

Twenty-four hours after surgical decompression, the patient regained alertness (GCS 14) and showed only a slight neurological deficit with an NIHSS of 5. Follow-up MRI showed additional acute stroke lesions in the left ACA territory, that had occurred perioperatively, but nevertheless the patient did well and was transferred to rehabilitation 3 weeks later.

Image findings

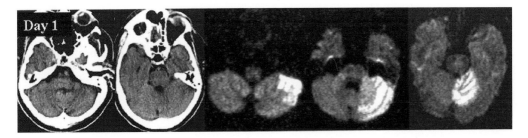

Figure 37.1 Day 1: Normal CT scan 6 hours after symptom onset shows no definite demarcation of ischemia, while diffusion-weighted MRI shortly thereafter shows acute ischemic lesion in the left cerebellar hemisphere.

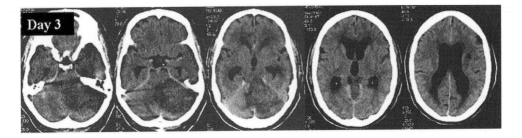

Figure 37.2 Day 3: Clinical deterioration is explained by the now obvious cerebellar lesion with brain stem compression by mass effect and compression of the cisterns around the brainstem and occlusion of the cerebral aqueduct causing hydrocephalus.

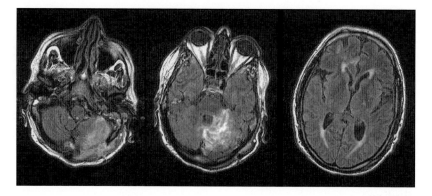

Figure 37.3 Postoperative MRI shows no mass effect in the posterior fossa and a normal ventricular system.

Diagnosis

Space-occupying cerebellar infarction treated by suboccipital craniectomy.

General remarks

The most common initial findings of acute cerebellar infarction include ataxia, vertigo, dysarthria, nausea, vomiting, difficulty sitting or standing without support, and a prominent headache. The clinical course in these patients may range from clinically stable neurological deficits to slow or very rapid deterioration; in some cases the patients initially present with coma. Patients with acute cerebellar stroke should therefore be best followed for up to 4 days in a neurologic intensive care setting with constant observation and frequent re-examination. Deterioration may be caused by direct mass effect of the lesion and brainstem compression or may be primarily explained by compression of the fourth ventricle and aqueduct with obstructive hydrocephalus. In the first instance, suboccipital craniectomy with evacuation of infarcted tissue is regarded as the best surgical approach; in cases with hydrocephalus ventriculostomy may be the only treatment required. American Heart Association Guidelines for spontaneous intracerebral hemorrhage management recommend surgical therapy in patients with cerebellar hemorrhage >3 cm who are neurologically deteriorating or who have brainstem compression and hydrocephalus from ventricular obstruction as soon as possible.

Special remarks

Studies concerning prognosis and prediction of deterioration are few. It has been shown that posterior inferior cerebellar artery territory infarcts with a triad of vertigo, headache, and gait imbalance at onset are more likely to deteriorate, while patients with superior cerebellar artery infarcts and predominate gait disturbance at onset usually have a more benign course. While it is clear that cerebellar infarction should be operated on as soon as progressive deterioration of consciousness develops – as performed in this case – the possible value of prophylactic ventriculostomy or decompression has not been evaluated.

CURRENT REVIEW

Jensen, M. B. & St Louis, E. K. Management of acute cerebellar stroke. *Arch. Neurol.* 2005; **62**:537–544.

SUGGESTED READING

Amarenco, P. The spectrum of cerebellar infarctions. *Neurology* 1991; **41**:973–979.

Auer, L. M., Auer, T., & Sayama, I. Indications for surgical treatment of cerebellar haemorrhage and infarction. *Acta Neurochir.* (Wien). 1986; **79**:74–79.

Broderick, J. P., Adams, H. P. Jr., Barsan, W. *et al.* Guidelines for the management of spontaneous intracerebral hemorrhage: a statement for healthcare professionals from a special writing group of the Stroke Council, American Heart Association. *Stroke* 1999; **30**:905–915.

Chaves, C. J., Caplan, L. R., Chung, C. S. *et al.* Cerebellar infarcts in the New England Medical Center Posterior Circulation Stroke Registry. *Neurology* 1994; **44**:1385–1390.

Kase, C. S., Norrving, B., Levine, S. R. *et al.* Cerebellar infarction. Clinical and anatomic observations in 66 cases. *Stroke* 1993; **24**:76–83.

Small problem with severe consequences

Clinical history

An 18-year-old girl presented initially to an ENT specialist in a private practice because of local inflammation on the right side of her face, after she manipulated a small furuncle at the right lateral aspect of her nose. She was sent to a regional hospital for systemic antibiotic treatment, which was started with penicillin, and the following day changed to sulfamethoxazole, trimethoprim, and cefuroxime. She was transferred to our hospital for further evaluation and intensive care treatment, 48 hours after onset of symptoms because of a rapidly progressive headache and decreased consciousness.

Examination

On admission, the patient was febrile, stuporous with intermittent phases of agitation, scoring 7 points on the Glasgow Coma Scale. On ophthalmologic examination marked proptosis, massive chemosis, and periorbital edema bilaterally, but more prominent on the right side, was noted. Pupils showed no reaction to light, the right pupil diameter was 3.5 mm, the left pupil diameter 7 mm; intraocular pressure was severely elevated. Extraocular movements were limited more on the left side. Meningeal signs were not noted. There was slight weakness of her left arm, pyramidal signs were negative. The remainder of her medical and neurological examination was normal.

Neurological scores

NIH not applicable; Barthel Index 0; GCS 7.

Special studies

Laboratory data were significant for a slight leukocytosis (8000 cells/mm^3), an elevated C-reactive protein of 290 mg/l, and signs of moderate consumptive coagulopathy. Her CSF indicated a bacterial meningoencephalitis with a marked neutrophilic pleocytosis with 1333 cells/mm^3 and a total protein of 2852 mg/l. Blood cultures revealed staphylococcus aureus sepsis, CSF culture was negative. Initial CT scan showed hyperdense superior ophthalmic veins bilaterally with signs of slight brain edema.

On follow-up neuroimaging with CT on day 4, the cavernous sinus was hyperdense bilaterally, indicative of thrombosis. Subsequently, on day 12, CT showed contrast enhancement in the right temporo-parietal region and the left hemisphere of the cerebellum compatible with abscesses. In summary, cranial CTs showed bilateral cavernous sinus thrombosis with thromboses of both superior orbital veins and abscesses in the right cerebral hemisphere and left cerebellum.

Follow-up

The clinical course of our patient was complicated by pneumonia with lung abscesses. She then developed respiratory failure and needed mechanical ventilation. *Staphylococcus aureus* sepsis was treated with the combination of ceftriaxone, vancomycin, and penicillin. Signs of septicemia, consumption coagulopathy and massive inflammatory response regressed during 10 days. Extubation on day 14 was followed by ventricular tachycardia and ventricular fibrillation followed by immediate cardiopulmonary resuscitation. After tracheostomy on day 22, the patient breathed spontaneously; 5 days later the tracheostomy was operatively occluded.

On neurological examination, besides marked slowing of behavior and thinking, she had a left third nerve palsy, brisker deep tendon reflexes on the left, and impaired fine motor skills on the left. The ophthalmologic examination showed improving direct and indirect pupillary reactions on the right with absent responses on the left side. Visual acuity was severely impaired on both sides with the patient only being able to count fingers at 2 feet (20/4000). Elevated intraocular pressures improved after treatment with mannitol and diamox. Antibiotic treatment was stopped at day 30, the patient being free from signs of septicemia, afebrile, with negative blood cultures. She was discharged to a rehabilitation unit.

Eighteen months later, we saw the patient again after a first generalized seizure. She reported two previous focal sensory seizures and was treated with lamotrigine. At that time, visual acuity had markedly improved (20/80 bilaterally), she planned professional training and was functioning independently with normal activities of daily living.

Image findings

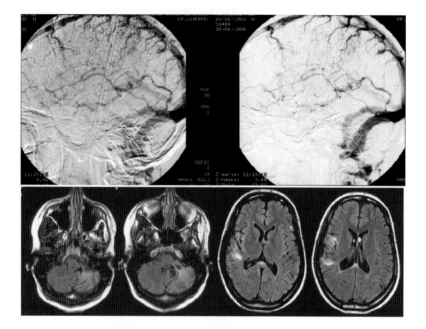

Figure 38.1 *Upper row*: Venous phase of cerebral angiography of the left internal carotid artery shows normal filling of the superior sagittal sinus and the transverse sinuses but poor contrast in the cavernous sinus. *Bottom row*: T_2-weighted FLAIR MRI performed after rehabilitation treatment shows residual hyperintense lesions in the left cerebellum and the right hemisphere.

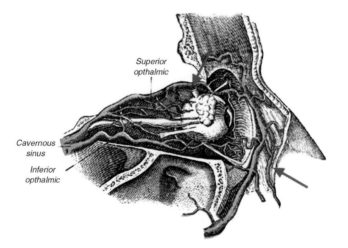

Figure 38.2 Arrows and dotted line indicate the posited route of transportation of infectious agents from facial veins to the cavernous sinus. Illustration modified after: Gray, H. *Anatomy of the Human Body*. Philadelphia: Lea & Febiger, 1918; Bartleby.com, 2000.

Diagnosis

Septic thrombosis of the cavernous sinuses, septic encephalitis with brain abscesses. Pneumonia with lung abscesses.

General remarks

Septic thrombosis of the cavernous sinuses or CST is a rare, though dramatic and potentially lethal illness, that may occur as a complication of infectious and noninfectious processes. CST most commonly follows infections of the middle third of the face ("muzzle area") due to *Staphylococcus aureus*. Bacteria entering the facial vein and pterygoid plexus from these sites may be carried to the cavernous sinus through the ophthalmic veins.

Other antecedent sites of infection include paranasal (usually sphenoid) sinusitis, dental abscess and, less often, otitis media. Fever is a nearly constant finding, but headache may not be prominent. Periorbital edema, chemosis, proptosis, and limitation of extraocular movements (especially lateral gaze) develop in almost all recognized cases. Involvement of the opposite eye frequently appears within 2 days following the onset of unilateral signs. Although computed tomography may be helpful, magnetic resonance imaging is probably the diagnostic procedure of choice. Before the availability of antibiotic treatment, mortality was near 100%, but it markedly decreased to approximately 20% to 30% during the era of antimicrobial agents. Treatment includes appropriate antibiotics and, often, surgical drainage of the primary focus of infection. Less than half of the patients recover completely, blindness is a severe sequel of the condition. The mortality rate is approximately 30% which makes it necessary to recognize, diagnose, and treat CST as soon as possible to minimize risks to the patient. Anticoagulants as an adjunctive therapeutic measure are controversially discussed, although a recent review suggests beginning anticoagulation after excluding hemorrhagic sequelae of CST radiologically.

FIRST DESCRIPTIONS

Duncan, A. *Contribution to Morbid Anatomy.* Edinburgh, 1821; 17,334.

Smith, D. Cavernous sinus thrombosis with notes of five cases. *Arch. Ophthalmol.* 1918; **47**:482–493.

Vigla, E. N. De la Morve Aigue chez l'homme. Theses de l'Ecole de Medecine, Paris, 1839.

CURRENT REVIEW

Ebright, J. R., Pace, M. T., & Niazi, A. F. Septic thrombosis of the cavernous sinuses. *Arch. Intern. Med.* 2001; **161**:2671–2676.

SUGGESTED READING

Arat, Y. O., Shetlar, D. J., & Rose, J. E. Blindness from septic thrombophlebitis of the orbit and cavernous sinus caused by *Fusobacterium nucleatum*. *Arch. Ophthalmol.* 2004; **122**:652–654.

Bhatia, K. & Jones, N. S. Septic cavernous sinus thrombosis secondary to sinusitis: are anticoagulants indicated? A review of the literature. *J. Laryngol. Otol.* 2002; **116**:667–676.

DiNubile, M. J. Septic thrombosis of the cavernous sinuses. *Arch. Neurol.* 1988; **45**:567–572.

Ellie, E., Houang, B., Louail, C. *et al.* CT and high-field MRI in septic thrombosis of the cavernous sinuses. *Neuroradiology* 1992; **34**:22–24.

Heckmann, J. G. & Tomandl, B. Cavernous sinus thrombosis. *Lancet* 2003; **362**:1958.

Sanchez, T. G. Cahali, M. B., Murakami, M. S., Butugan, O., & Miniti, A. Septic thrombosis of orbital vessels due to cutaneous nasal infection. *Am J. Rhinol.* 1997; **11**:429–433.

Schuknecht, B., Simmen, D., Yuksel, C., & Valavanis, A. Tributary venosinus occlusion and septic cavernous sinus thrombosis: CT and MR findings. *Am. J. Neuroradiol.* 1998; **19**:617–626.

Southwick, F. S., Richardson, E. P. Jr., & Swartz, M. N. Septic thrombosis of the dural venous sinuses. *Medicine (Baltimore)* 1986; **65**:82–106.

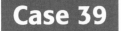

Dizzy spells and double vision

Clinical history

A 72-year-old woman reported sudden attacks of dizziness, facial numbness and double vision.

General history

She was treated for hypertension, and diabetes mellitus during the past 10 years.

Examination

Neurological examination showed a complex eye movement abnormality consisting of an incomplete right internuclear ophthalmoplegia, suppression of vertical optokinetic nystagmus, and skew deviation. Gait ataxia was also noted.

Neurological scores on admission

NIH 1; Barthel Index 100; GCS 15.

Special studies

Axial MRI through the posterior fossa showed a hemorrhagic pontine lesion extending dorsally to the floor of the fourth ventricle consistent with a cavernoma without any associated venous malformation.

Follow-up

As edema surrounding the lesion on MRI slightly increased the following day, the patient's symptoms were slightly progressive. One week later she had surgery using a suboccipital medial transventricular approach to remove the cavernoma. The patient did well with only residual intermittent nausea and returned home soon after operation.

Image findings

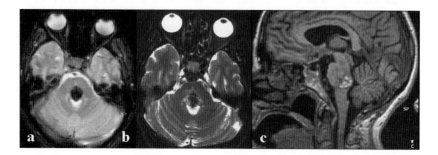

Figure 39.1 (a) T_2^*-susceptibility weighted, (b) T_2-weighted and (c) non-contrast T_1-weighted MRI showing a cavernoma of the pons.

Diagnosis

Acute hemorrhage of the pons due to cavernous malformation.

General remarks

Cavernous angiomas, or cavernomas of the central nervous system, are lesions that consist of blood-filled cavities lined by a single layer of endothelium and separated by neuroglia but not by neural tissue. Prevalence estimates from autopsy series vary from 0.39 % to 0.9%.

Cavernous malformations can be located anywhere in the body, including the liver, rectum, kidney, eyes, nerves, spinal cord, and brain. Cerebral cavernous angioma malformations can be inherited as an autosomal dominant condition or arise de novo. Cerebral cavernous malformations are usually supratentorial but can occur anywhere in the neural axis and have been described in the brainstem, spinal cord, lateral ventricle and the cavernous sinus. Cranial radiation, coexistent vascular malformation, genetic and hormonal factors, and previous surgery for intracranial lesions have been described as risk factors for cavernomas.

The natural history of brainstem cavernomas indicate a high risk of rupture, bleeding and significant morbidity. There is also a slight propensity to rebleeding. However, in a series of 37 patients cavernomas less than 10 mm in diameter, there was a relatively low risk of rebleeding.

Special remarks

Direct treatment of brain stem cavernomas represent a considerable challenge due to the close proximity of the vital structures in the skull base. However, more recently surgical treatment has been achieved with acceptable morbidity and mortality and excellent results have been reported by several groups. Imaging developments aided by microsurgical techniques have improved the ability to deal with these lesions.

SUGGESTED READING

Kupersmith, M. J., Kalish, H., Epstein, F. *et al.* Natural history of brainstem cavernous malformations. *Neurosurgery* 2001; **48**:47–53; discussion 53–54.

Mathiesen, T., Edner, G., & Kihlström, L. Deep and brainstem cavernomas: a consecutive 8-years series. *J. Neurosurg.* 2003; **99**:31–7.

Ogilvy, C. S., Stieg, P. E., Awad, I. *et al.* Recommendations for the management of intracranial arteriovenous malformations: a statement for healthcare professionals from a special writing group of the Stroke Council, American Stroke Association. *Circulation* 2001; **103**:2644–2657.

Rabinstein, A. A., Tisch, S. H., Clelland, R. L., & Wijdicks, E. F. Cause is the main predictor of outcome in patients with pontine hemorrhage. *Cerebrovasc. Dis.* 2004; **17**:66–71.

Sandalcioglu, I. E., Wiedemayer, H., Secer, S., Asgari, S., & Stolke, D. Surgical removal of brain stem cavernous malformations: surgical indications, technical considerations, and results. *J. Neurol. Neurosurg. Psychiatry* 2002; **72**:351–355.

Case 40

Bad disease with good outcome

Clinical history

A 69-year-old man reported multiple transient episodes characterized by loss of strength in the left arm and slurred speech lasting less than 30 minutes during the last 3 days.

General history

He had a 5-year history of coronary heart disease and hypertension.

Examination

Neurologic examination on admission was normal.

Neurological scores

NIH 0; Barthel Index 100; GCS 15.

Special studies

Ultrasound duplex examination showed a high grade stenosis at the vertebrobasilar junction. He continued with further transient ischemic attacks for the following 2 days despite a sufficient PTT-controlled anticoagulation with heparin. On day 3 he developed a tetraparesis and brainstem signs (inability to swallow, aspiration, dysfunction of respiration). He became comatose within 4 hours and was admitted to the ICU for artificial ventilation. Angiography, ultrasound, and MRI showed an occlusion of the basilar artery. MRI at this point showed acute pontine and cerebellar infarction. Thrombolysis was not performed because of the long time window (2 days) and because of the extended brainstem lesions. The patient was treated for complications (pneumonia, sepsis, bradycardia) but did not receive further anticoagulation or any other specific therapy. He remained ventilated for another 3 weeks and after a prolonged extubation time he showed severe ataxia, complete inability to swallow, a severe tetraparesis and a complex oculomotor disturbance. Although the basilar artery remained occluded, neurological as well as functional scores improved.

Follow-up

The patient became completely independent within 5 months and remained stable without further cerebrovascular events for the next 5 years despite permanent occlusion of the basilar artery.

Image findings

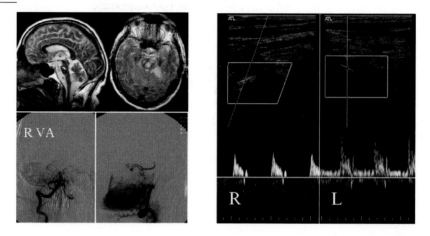

Figure 40.1 *Left*: T$_2$-weighted MRI showing multiple pontine and left cerebellar ischemic lesions. Conventional angiography below shows no filling of the basilar artery, only minimal flow in the distal left vertebral artery and collateral flow mainly from the right PICA. *Right*: High resistance flow pattern in both vertebral arteries R > L indicating distal vessel pathology.

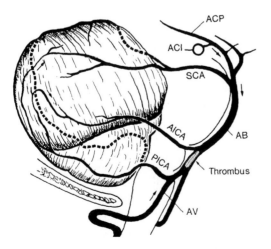

Figure 40.2 Illustration of the posterior arterial circulation of the brain. AB: basilar artery (with thrombus), ACI: internal carotid artery, ACP: posterior cerebellar artery, AICA: anterior inferior cerebellar artery, AV: vertebral artery, PICA: posterior inferior cerebellar artery, SCA: superior cerebellar artery (adapted from L. Caplan).

Diagnosis

Persistent basilar artery occlusion with good recovery after initial coma and mechanical ventilation.

General remarks

The first basilar artery occlusion was reported in 1868 by Hayem. Kubik and Adams' classic report in 1946 shaped modern concepts of basilar artery disease. They concluded that basilar artery occlusions are characterized by frequent early loss of consciousness, common bilateral involvement, and combinations of pupillary abnormalities, ocular and other cranial nerve palsies, dysarthria, extensor plantar reflexes, hemiplegia or quadriplegia. Description of amnesia, hemianopia, and other posterior cerebral artery manifestations were added some years later. In situ atherosclerosis and cardioembolism are the most common causes of basilar artery strokes. Less frequent etiologies include dissection, migraine, dolichoectasia, vasculitis, and paradoxical embolism.

Special remarks

In the past, basilar artery occlusion was regarded as a disease with extremely poor prognosis, often diagnosed with absolute certainty only at autopsy. The advent of fast, reliable and non-invasive vascular imaging techniques such as ultrasound, as well as CT and MR angiography, has made diagnosis of basilar artery occlusion possible in patients with severe neurological deficits as well as in patients with limited ischemic injury and therefore, a more benign prognosis. In cases diagnosed early and treated quickly with thrombolysis and endovascular therapy, survival rate may be increased and disability limited.

The long-term risk of recurrent TIA or stroke after first ischemic presentation of basilar artery occlusion disease is poorly defined. In a review of the medical records of 25 patients admitted into the intensive care unit with a clinical diagnosis of acute basilar artery occlusion and need for mechanical ventilation, no neurological improvement beyond a locked-in syndrome occurred in survivors. The presented patient had a favorable 3-year follow-up. Despite continuous basilar artery occlusion on ultrasound and MRA, the patient recovered from coma within 3 months and improved to a slight dysfunctional impairment within a year and did well for the next 4 years without any new cerebrovascular event. Whether or not endovascular stenting and angioplasty is beneficial or harmful in unstable conditions has not been evaluated and is a matter of controversy based on case reports only amongst neurologists, interventional neuroradiologists and stroke physicians.

FIRST DESCRIPTION

Hayem, M. G. Sur la thrombose par arterite du tronc basilaire. Comme cause du mort rapide. *Arch. Physiol. Norm. Pathol.* 1868; **1**:270–289.

CURRENT REVIEW

Voetsch, B., DeWitt, L. D., Pessin, M. S., & Caplan, L. R. Basilar artery occlusive disease in the New England Medical Center Posterior Circulation Registry. *Arch. Neurol.* 2004; **61**:496–504.

SUGGESTED READING

Brandt, T. 'Diagnosis and thrombolytic therapy of acute basilar artery occlusion: a review.' *Clin. Exp. Hypertens.* 2002; **24**:611–622.

Ferbert, A., Bruckmann, H., & Drummen, R. Clinical features of proven basilar artery occlusion. *Stroke* 1990; **21**:1135–1142.

Horowitz, M., Jovin, T., Levy, E., & Anderson, W. Emergent basilar artery and bilateral posterior cerebral artery angioplasty, urokinase thrombolysis, and stenting for acute basilar artery occlusion secondary to diagnostic cardiac catheterization: case presentation. *J. Neuroimaging* 2005; **15**:315–318.

Straube, T., Stingele, R., & Jansen, O. Primary stenting of intracranial atherosclerotic stenoses. *Cardiovasc. Intervent. Radiol.* 2005; **28**:289–295.

Wijdicks, E. F. & Scott, J. P. Outcome in patients with acute basilar artery occlusion requiring mechanical ventilation. *Stroke* 1996; **27**:1301–1303.

Livid skin and stroke

Clinical history

A 48-year-old woman described a non-specific feeling of weakness, headache and slight word finding difficulties during the preceding 5 days. She was a smoker, and had several vascular risk factors with a 5-year history of arterial hypertension and hypercholesterolemia.

General history

Uterine myomas and hysterectomy 5 years earlier; ovarectomy due to multiple cysts 2 months earlier. She received oral estradiol substitution. There was no family history of neurologic disease. There was no family history of neurologic or other diseases.

Examination

Neurological examination showed a slight right-sided brachial paresis with increased muscle tone. Neuropsychological testing found moderate verbal and visual memory deficits, decreased word fluency and speed of reading as well as slowed color naming. On general physical examination, the skin over her knees and elbows had a patchy blue–red discoloration.

Neurological scores

NIH 2; Barthel Index 100; GCS 15.

Special studies

Transcranial ultrasound showed a moderate stenosis of the left proximal MCA (max velocity 160 cm/s). Diffusion-weighted MRI showed multiple acute ischemic lesions in the left MCA territory, while FLAIR images revealed multiple contralateral chronic lesions – all of which had an embolic pattern with mainly cortical involvement.

The following was found on extensive autoimmunological laboratory analysis: elevated titer of antinuclear-antibodies (1:1280), postitive ss-DNA-antibodies (96 RE/ml), positive IgM cardiolipin antibodies (11 MRL/U/ml) and positive ds-DNA-antibodies (ELISA). Skin biopsy showed lymphohistiocytic perivascular dermatitis without any other significant histological alterations. There was no evidence of livedo vasculitis, findings were, however, consistent with livedo racemosa.

Follow-up

A diagnosis of stroke due to Sneddon's syndrome was made and oral anti-coagulation with phenprocoumon was initiated. After a period of rehabilitation, she fully recovered. She was treated with aspirin for secondary stroke prevention. There were no further cerebrovascular events.

Image findings

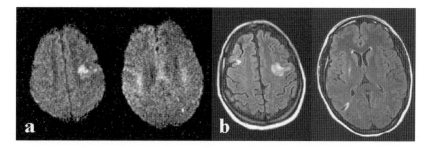

Figure 41.1 (a) Multiple cortical acute ischemic lesions in the left MCA territory on diffusion-weighted MRI. (b) T_2-weighted FLAIR images show chronic cortical lesions and a discrete lesion in the external capsule in the right MCA territory.

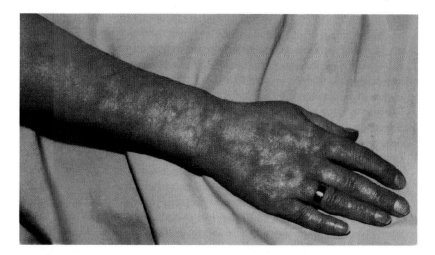

Figure 41.2 Typical fixed, patchy, net-like violaceous skin discoloration of livedo racemosa.

Diagnosis

Stroke due to Sneddon's syndrome.

General remarks

In 1965 the British dermatologist, Ian Bruce Sneddon, described six patients with livedo reticularis and cerebrovascular episodes. This clinical presentation became known as Sneddon's syndrome although five years before, Champion and Rook had reported a similar case and even in 1907 Ehrmann had already described a patient with syphilis and stroke in association with livedo racemosa.

The Sneddon syndrome is generally considered an arteriopathy of small- and medium-sized vessels of unknown origin. Pathohistological findings in skin biopsies are various and often normal. Wohlrab *et al.* found intimal proliferation with occlusion of arterioles and migration of medial smooth muscle cells in 12 of 15 patients and showed that sensitivity of skin biopsy could be augmented up to 80% by obtaining three repeated biopsies. The lack of homologous pathological data from brain and cerebral vessels makes it difficult to understand the pathogenesis of stroke in this syndrome. Antiphospholipid antibodies are frequently associated suggesting autoimmunological genesis of Sneddon's syndrome. Clinical manifestations are livedo reticularis and ischemic stroke particularly in the MCA-territory, but occasionally accompanying episodes of migraine, headache, transient ischemic attacks, dizziness, or vascular dementia are reported. Cardiac or renal involvement may occur. Reasonable diagnostic evaluation in addition to clinical examination (especially looking for peripheral embolic lesions, retinal embolic material, joint involvement, skin lesions), should include neuroimaging studies (extra- and intracranial ultrasound, cranial MRI/MRA and cerebral angiography if indicated), extended laboratory studies (including APL, lupus anticoagulant, anticardiolipin antibodies, β-2 glycoprotein-1 antibodies, VDRL, platelet count, hematocrit, coagulation parameters, antinuclear antigen, rheumatoid factors, serum protein electrophoresis, cryoglobulins, circulating immune complexes, purified protein electrophoresis, and skin biopsy). As no specific test for Sneddon's syndrome exists so far, differential diagnosis from collagen vascular diseases, infectious diseases, metabolic disorders, neoplasm, cryoglobulinemia may be difficult.

Current treatment of patients with Sneddon's syndrome is still controversial and experimental, differing between two subgroups of APL-positive and -negative Sneddon's syndrome. APL-positive Sneddon's syndrome patients may be treated like primary antiphospholipid syndrome whereas in APL-negative Sneddon's syndrome, antiplatelet therapy might be as effective as high-dose warfarin.

Special remarks

The differential diagnosis of antiphospholipid syndrome was considered in our patient, who had anticardiolipin antibodies and a history of thrombocytopenia. A diagnosis of systemic lupus erythematodes might also be entertained, because of additionally positive ANA and ds-DNA antibodies. Existing arterial hypertension, nicotine abuse, and estrogen substitution can be regarded as known triggers for SNS. Family history of SNS is rare but suggests autosomal dominant pattern of inheritance, with incomplete penetrance.

FIRST DESCRIPTION

Champion, R. H. & Rook, A. Livedo reticularis. *Proc. Roy. Soc. Med.* 1960; **53**:961.

Ehrmann, S. Ein neues Gefaesssymptom bei Lues. *Wien. Medi. Wochenschri* 1907; **57**:777–782.

Sneddon, I. B. Cerebrovascular lesions and livedo reticularis. *Br. J. Dermatol.* 1965; **77**:180–185.

SUGGESTED READING

Floel, A., Imai, T., Lohmann, H., Bethke, F., Sunderkoetter, C., & Droste, D. W. Therapy of Sneddon Syndrome. *Eur. Neurol.* 2002; **48**:126–132.

Frances, C., Papo, T., Wechsler, B., Laporte, J. L., Biousse, V., & Piette, J. C. Sneddon syndrome with or without antiphospholipid antibodies. A comparative study in 46 patients. *Medicine (Baltimore)* 1999; **78**:209–219.

Frances, C. & Piette, J. C. The mystery of Sneddon syndrome: relationship with antiphospholipid syndrome and sytemic lupus erythematosus. *J. Autoimmun.* 2000; **15**:139–143.

Rautenberg, W., Hennerici, M., Aulich, A., Holzke, E., & Lakomek, H. J. Immunosuppressive therapy and Sneddon's syndrome. *Lancet* 1988; **2**:629–630.

Stockhammer, G., Felber, S. R., Zelger, B. *et al.* Sneddon's syndrome: diagnosis by skin biospy and MRI in 17 patients. *Stroke* 1993; **24**:685–690.

Szmyrka-Kaczmarek, M., Daikeler, T., Benz, D. & Koetter, I. Familial inflammatory Sneddon's syndrome-case report and review of the literature. *Clin. Rheumatol.* 2005; **24**:79–82.

Wohlrab, J., Fischer, M., Wolter, M., & Marsch, W. C. Diagnostic impact and sensitivity of skin biopsies in Sneddon's syndrome. A report of 15 cases. *Br. J. Dermatol.* 2001; **145**:285–288.

Stroke mimicking vestibular neuronitis

Clinical history

A 33-year-old man was admitted to the otolaryngology clinic due to intense rotatory vertigo, nausea and sweating, and spontaneous nystagmus since several days with the diagnosis of vestibular neuronitis. After normal caloric testing, but persistent symptoms of vertigo and nausea accompanied by neck pain, a neurologist was consulted.

Examination

Neurological examination showed spontaneous bilateral nystagmus without further focal neurological signs, hearing loss, tinnitus or meningism. The patient described circumscribed bilateral neck pain. He recalled a minor go-cart accident 2 weeks before.

Neurological scores

NIH 0; Barthel Index 100; GCS 15.

Special studies

While initial CCT was normal, Doppler/duplex examination showed hyperpulsatile flow in the left VA and a circumscribed non-echogenic thickening of the vessel wall in the right VA on B-mode scan consistent with a mural hematoma. Subsequent MRI examination confirmed the mural hematoma in the proximal V1/2-segments of the right VA and a long-segment dissection of the left distal VA.

Follow-up

Two days later, while taking secondary prophylaxis with low-dose heparin, the patient developed sudden dysarthria and a right hemiparesis. Diffusion-weighted imaging showed multiple acute ischemic lesion in the left PICA territory.

No further ischemic events occurred and the patient was independent after a rehabilitation therapy. After his discharge, he was treated with aspirin and, in a follow-up MRI performed 1 year later, both VA had fully recanalized.

Image findings

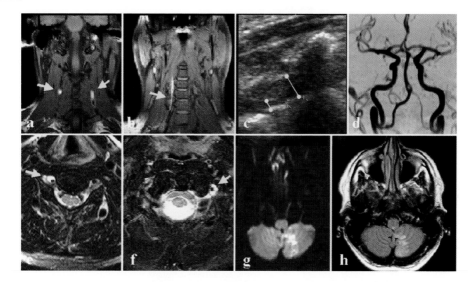

Figure 42.1 (a), (b) Yellow arrows point to T_1-hyperintense signal along the course of the vertebral arteries indicating mural hematoma in coronal slices. (c) Ultrasound B-mode scan shows a circumscribed non-echogenic thickening of the vessel wall in the left VA consistent with a mural hematoma. (d) On TOF-MRA of the intracranial vessels the left distal VA is poorly contrasted, while the distal portion of the right VA appears normal. (e), (f) Transverse slices show hyperintense semicircular mural hematoma of both VA. (g), (h) Diffusion-weighted and T_2-weighted FLAIR sequences show acute ischemic lesion in the left PICA territory.

Diagnosis

Hemodynamic bilateral vertebral artery dissection with delayed embolic stroke.

General remarks

Although vertebral artery dissection is an uncommon vascular disorder (more rarely seen than dissection of the carotid artery), it is an important cause of posterior circulation ischemia in young patients (<45 years), accounting for about 10% to 20% of these cases. The estimated annual incidence is 1 to 1.5 per 100 000.

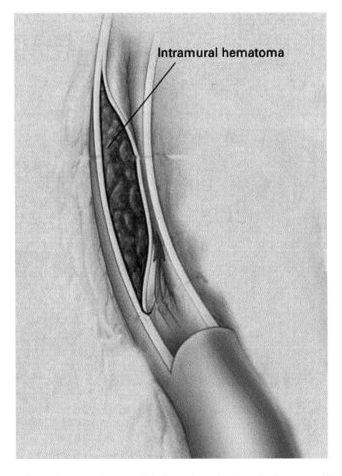

Intramural hematoma

Figure 42.2 Schematic view of an arterial dissection, showing the intramural hematoma with occlusion of the vessel lumen.

Precipitating events associated with a hyperextension of the neck are common in cervical artery dissections and may damage the arterial vessel wall due to mechanical stretching. Spinal manipulative therapy has also been shown to be associated with vertebral arterial dissection. Typical symptoms are neck pain and headache, the latter most often in the occipital area in the first stage due to pain fiber stimulation, while later embolism from focal thrombosis or aneurysms may be threatening.

Special remarks

In our patient a minor go-cart accident might have been linked to the development of vertebral artery dissection. Although classically only a short interval between dissection and consequent stroke is assumed, in VA dissections the time course from hemodynamic encroachment to presentation with an ischemic event may be considerably longer than previously recognized and may range from a few minutes to several weeks.

FIRST DESCRIPTION

Fisher, C. M., Ojemann, R. G., & Robertson, G. H. Spontaneous dissection of the cervico-cerebral arteries. *Can. J. Neurol. Sci.* 1978; **5**:9–19.

CURRENT REVIEW

Caplan, L. R. & Biousse, V. Cervicocranial arterial dissections. *J. Neuroophthalmol.* 2004; **24**:299–305.

SUGGESTED READING

Caplan, L. R., Zarins, C. K., & Hemmatti, M. Spontaneous dissection of the extracranial vertebral arteries. *Stroke* 1985; **16**:1030–1038.

Caso, V., Paciaroni, M., Corea, F. *et al.* Recanalization of cervical artery dissection: influencing factors and role in neurological outcome. *Cerebrovasc. Dis.* 2004; **17**:93–97.

Mas, J. L., Henin, D., Bousser, M. G., Chain, F., & Hauw, J. J. Dissecting aneurysm of the vertebral artery and cervical manipulation: a case report with autopsy. *Neurology* 1989; **39**:512–515.

Nazir, F. S. & Muir, K. W. Prolonged interval between vertebral artery dissection and ischemic stroke. *Neurology* 2004; **62**:1646–1647.

Smith, W. S., Johnston, S. C., Skalabrin, E. J. *et al.* Spinal manipulative therapy is an independent risk factor for vertebral artery dissection. *Neurology* 2003; **60**:1424–1428.

Tettenborn, B., Caplan, L. R., Sloan, M. A. *et al.* Postoperative brainstem and cerebellar infarcts. *Neurology* 1993; **43**:471–477.

Scuba diver with decompression sickness

Clinical history

A 51-year-old engineer and recreational diving instructor with an experience of more than 1300 scuba dives had repeatedly developed slight symptoms of DCS after scuba diving within the last 10 years presenting with exanthema, pruritus, and arthralgia. These symptoms were transient and occurred after "normal" dives, without violation of decompression rules.

Otherwise, his past medical history was normal. He is a non-smoker with normal body weight (BMI 23) and no vascular risk factors.

Examination

Neurological examination was normal.

Neurological scores

NIH 0; Barthel Index 100; GCS 15.

Special studies

As a voluntary participant at a research project, he underwent a screening test for persistent foramen ovale, that was performed by means of echocontrast-enhanced TCD monitoring before and after a Valsalva maneuver. We also performed cranial MRI. The TCD-based persistent foramen ovale test revealed a significant right-to-left shunt with detection of high intensity signals in the arterial circulation spontaneously and after Valsalva maneuver. This finding was then confirmed by transesophageal echocardiography, which showed a significant persistent foramen ovale III° with crossover of contrast agent bubbles from the right to the left atrium, but no atrial aneurysm. MRI showed multiple tiny T_2-hyperintense lesions in the deep white matter of both hemispheres.

Image findings

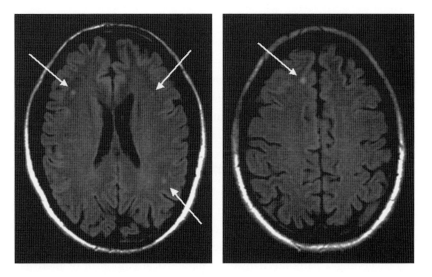

Figure 43.1 FLAIR (fluid attenuated inversion recovery) transversal MRI images show multiple tiny lesions in the deep white matter of both hemispheres (arrows). Lesions were hyperintense also on T_2- and proton-density-weighted sequences (not shown).

Diagnosis

Cerebral white matter lesions in a recreational scuba diver with large PFO.

General remarks

Recreational scuba ("self-contained underwater breathing apparatus") diving is a very popular sport with approximately 1.5 million certified divers in Germany, and six million in the United States. Scuba diving involves a risk for neurologic injuries caused by decompression sickness, arterial gas embolism, anoxia, and the toxic effects of high partial pressure of breathing gases. The medical problems of divers caused by DCS are based upon the phenomenon of emerging and expanding inert gas bubbles during the ascent phase of a scuba dive. Symptoms associated with DCS are commonly due to local tissue damage and may range from slight and reversible signs of exanthema, pruritus, rash, subcutaneous edema or arthralgia, to severe and potentially life-threatening affection of the lung or the central nervous system. Another severe manifestation of decompression injuries develops due to arterial gas embolism, where a rupture of alveoli in the lung with consecutive access of gas bubbles into the arterial circulation leads to acute generalized embolic disease.

Special remarks

The pathogenesis of DCS symptoms after "normal" dives with regular ascent velocity is more complex. In venous blood, inert gas bubbles are known to be present already after ascents from shallow water depths. However, since intact lungs are a competent filter for these bubbles, they usually do not enter the arterial circulation. Therefore, a right-to-left-shunt, in particular a persistent foramen ovale has been proposed as potential pathway for venous gas bubbles, particular under conditions of increased intra-thoracic pressure. The prevalence of persistent foramen ovale has been found to be increased in divers with DCS. Asymptomatic brain lesions on MRI have been found to be more frequent in sport divers than in non-diving controls. Multiple brain lesions were shown to be significantly associated with the presence of a large persistent foramen ovale, suggesting a pathomechanism of paradoxical embolism of inert gas bubbles to contribute to the development of cerebral white matter lesions in divers.

SUGGESTED READING

Brubakk, A. & Neuman, T. (ed.) *Bennett and Elliotts' Physiology and Medicine of Diving.* 5th edn., W. B. Saunders, 2003.

Knauth, M., Ries, S., Pohlmann, S. *et al.* Cohort study of multiple brain lesions in sport divers: role of a patent foramen ovale. *Br. Med. J.* 1997; **314**:701–705.

Moon, R. E., Camporesi, E. M., & Kisslo, J. A. Patent foramen ovale and decompression sickness in divers. *Lancet* 1989; **1**:513–514.

Reul, J., Weis, J., Jung, A., Willmes, K., & Thron, A. Central nervous system lesions and cervical disc herniations in amateur divers. *Lancet* 1995; **345**:1403–1405.

Ries, S., Knauth, M., Kern, R. *et al.* Arterial gas embolism after decompression: correlation with right-to-left shunting *Neurology* 1999; **52**:401–404.

Wilmshurst, P. T., Byrne, J. C., & Webb-Peploe, M. M. Relation between intraatrial shunts and decompression sickness in divers. *Lancet* 1989; **2**:1302–1305.

Memory loss after gastrointestinal endoscopy

Clinical history

A 65-year-old woman presented for upper gastrointestinal endoscopy. For preparation a topical, local anesthetic (Xylocain-spray) was sprayed into the pharynx. Endoscopy was performed in anteflexion of the head. As the patient wanted to drive home after upper gastrointestinal endoscopy, no sedation was used. The patient tolerated the procedure well and a gastric ulcer of 1 cm in diameter was found (Grade Forrest III), and histologically a *Helicobacter pylori* infection was proven. Afterwards, the patient was unaware of why she was in hospital. This alarmed the surgeons performing the endoscopy, especially since no premedication had been given.

General history

Gastric reflux.

Examination

The patient was unable to acquire or remember new information or recall the near past (the last 2 years) without psychomotor slowing or loss of personal identity. The findings on further neurological examination were normal.

Neurological scores

NIH 0; Barthel Index 80; GCS 15.

Special studies

Under the assumption of a TGA serial MRI was performed. Sixty minutes after symptom onset, no lesion was detectable. MRI was repeated after 24 and

48 hours, on the latter diffusions- und T$_2$-weighted images revealed an acute small hyperintense lesion in the anterior section of the left hippocampus.

Extensive stroke work-up could not identify high-grade vascular or cardiac risk factors.

Follow-up

Full clinical recovery was made after 6 hours.

Image findings

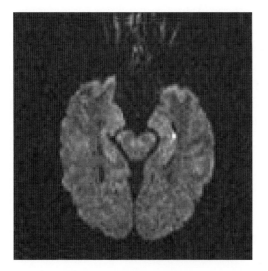

Figure 44.1 DWI hyperintense lesion in the anterior left hippocampus indicating cytotoxic edema.

Diagnosis

Transient global amnesia.

General remarks

There is still limited knowledge on the location and etiology of TGA. MR studies including DWI magnetic resonance imaging have recently been able to demonstrate consistently the location and therefore details of the underlying pathology of TGA. Of 31 patients studied, 26 developed a small, punctate DWI lesion in the lateral aspect of the hippocampal formation (pes and fimbria hippocampi) on either side (left $n = 15$, right $n = 6$) or bilaterally ($n = 5$). Lesions were rarely noted in the hyperacute phase ($n = 2$), but all became visible regularly at 48 h. While TGA remains pathophysiologically partly mysterious, the concept of delayed ischemic mechanisms being involved is appealing. High metabolic rates leading to relative hypoperfusion in the subcortical vascular borderzone in patients with mild vascular changes are known to be associated with delayed ischemic mechanisms. Similar processes occurring at a hippocampal level could be the natural history of sporadic transient global amnesia.

Special remarks

In the case presented, several precipitating factors for TGA can be identified: a Valsalva-manoever restricting cerebral venous drainage via superior cava vein, potentially triggering cardio-/arterialembolic mechanisms, but also the strong flexion of the head, potentially hindering free basilar blood flow. Whether – in the present case – there is any association apart from a temporal coincidence, is speculative.

FIRST DESCRIPTION

Fisher, C. M. & Adams, R. D. Transient global amnesia. *Trans. Am. Neurol. Assoc.* 1958; **83**:143–146.

CURRENT REVIEW

Pantoni, L., Lamassa, M., & Inzitari, D. Transient global amnesia: a review emphasizing pathogenetic aspects. *Acta Neurol. Scand.* 2000; **102**:275–283.

SUGGESTED READING

Gass, A., Gaa, J., Hirsch, J., Schwartz, A. & Hennerici, M. G. Lack of evidence of acute ischemic tissue change in transient global amnesia on single-shot echo-planar diffusion-weighted MRI. *Stroke* 1999; **30**:2070–2072.

Quinette, P., Guillery-Girard, B., Dayan, J. *et al.* What does transient global amnesia really mean? Review of the literature and thorough study of 142 cases. *Brain* 2006; **129**: 1640–1658.

Sander, D., Winbeck, K., Etgen, T., Knapp, R., Klingelhöfer, J., & Conrad, B. Disturbance of venous flow patterns in patients with transient global amnesia. *Lancet* 2000; **356**: 1982–1984.

Sedlaczek, O., Hirsch, J. G., Grips, E. *et al.* Detection of delayed focal MR changes in the lateral hippocampus in transient global amnesia. *Neurology* 2004; **62**:2165–2170.

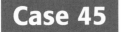

Case 45

Aphasia and severe headache

Clinical history

A 35-year-old woman arrived in the emergency room with suspected cerebral ischemia presenting with acute onset of global aphasia and fluctuating right-sided motor-sensory hemideficit since approximately 90 minutes. She reported nausea and dizziness. Medical history-taking was impossible, but family members said that she had been treated for cerebral ischemia in a hospital 4 years ago.

Examination

On neurologic examination, the patient had an obvious left hemispheric syndrome with global aphasia and fluctuating right-sided motor–sensory hemideficit and Babinski sign.

Neurological scores

NIH 5; Barthel Index 40; GCS 13.

Special studies

Because of the strongly fluctuating clinical symptoms, MRI instead of CT was performed prior to potential thrombolysis, revealing the unexpected finding of hypoperfusion of the complete left hemisphere on the TTP maps and the lack of an acute ischemic lesion more than 100 minutes after symptom onset. Within the following 6 hours, her symptoms resolved completely and the patient reported about strong throbbing fronto-nuchal headache. Now she could report having typical attacks of headache with and without aura since being a teenager; however, the diagnosis of migraine had not been made earlier. Attacks were not frequent and accompanying symptoms had never been this severe. She additionally described visual disturbances preceding the current attack. Further diagnostic testing revealed a significant right-to-left atrial shunt.

Image findings

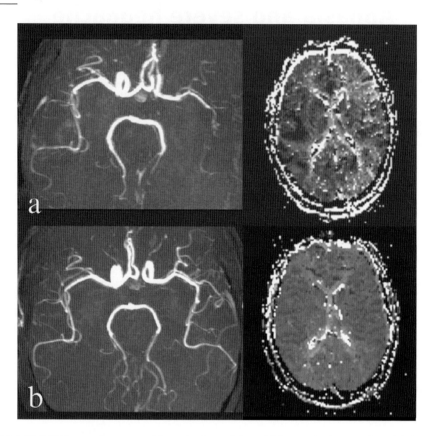

Figure 45.1 Initial MRA reveals asymmetric projection of the middle cerebral artery (MCA) left ≪ right and delayed contrast agent arrival in the left hemisphere on TTP maps – in all three vascular territories (a). On follow-up examination, angiography and PWI indicate normalization with symmetric perfusion (b).

Diagnosis

Complicated migraine with PFO.

General remarks

There are still numerous uncertainties about the pathophysiology of migraine with aura. The neuronal hypothesis suggests that aura symptoms are due to or at least associated with the development of a cortical spreading depression, which was shown in experimental studies to propagate at a similar speed as aura-associated symptoms. According to the "vascular hypothesis," the initial symptoms are attributed to an initial decrease in vascular diameter with reduced perfusion in the affected territory followed by hyperperfusion leading to headache. However, the initial blood flow reductions have been found to be marginal, unlikely to reach the oligemic/ischemic thresholds. Thus a causal relationship between low blood flow and functional failure remains difficult to understand. MR can visualize migraine with aura in different, clearly separated phases of blood flow and PWI while DWI lesions do not occur. In patients with acute onset of neurological deficits, the latter findings may be the only method of differentiating it from stroke. This is therapeutically relevant as the exclusion of manifest cerebral ischemia prevents unnecessary thrombolysis.

Special remarks

MRI findings in this case study show different, clearly separated phases of blood flow and perfusion. In the aura phase the patient was dysphasic and hypoperfusion may well have contributed to the patients clinical deficits. The hypoperfusion seen on MRI involved anterior and posterior circulation territories alike, that make other causes like transient embolic ischemia unlikely. The hypoperfusion was located mainly in cortical regions and less pronounced in the basal ganglia. The genetic disposition of migraine to PFO is well known.

FIRST DESCRIPTION

Willis, T. *The London Practice of Physick*: or the whole practical part of physick. Printed for Thomas Basset and William Cooke, London 1685; 386–387.

CURRENT REVIEW

Goadsby, P. B., Lipton, R. B., & Ferrai, M. D. Migraine: current understanding and management. *N. Engl. J. Med.* 2002; **346**:257–270.

SUGGESTED READING

Andersson, J. L., Muhr, C., Lilja, A., Valind, S., Lundberg, P. O., & Langstrom, B. Regional cerebral blood flow and oxygen metabolism during migraine with and without aura. *Cephalalgia* 1997; **17**:570–579.

Leao, A. Spreading depression of activity in the cerebral cortex; *J. Neurophysiol.* 1944; **7**:359–390.

Milner, P. M. Note on a possible correspondence between the scotomas of migraine and spreading depression of Leão. *EEG Clin. Neurophysiol.* 1958; **10**:705.

O'Brien, M. Cerebral blood changes in migraine. *Headache* 1971; **10**:139.

Olsen, S. T., Friberg, L., & Lassen, N. A. Ischemia may be the primary cause of the neurologic deficits in classic migraine. *Arch. Neurol.* 1987; **44**:156–161.

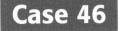

Case 46

Progressive neurological decline and fever

Clinical history

A previously healthy 42-year-old man gave a history of headache, dizziness, visual blurring, abnormal gait, and general exhaustion. He was referred to Neurology after brain imaging performed in a radiology practice had raised a suspicion of multiple sclerosis. Except for migraine with aura since adolescence, there was no relevant past medical history.

Examination

Initial neurological examination showed brisk deep tendon reflexes but was otherwise normal.

Neurological scores on admission

NIH 0; Barthel Index 100; GCS 15.

Special studies

A significant CSF pleocytosis with 48 cells/mm^3 with predominant lymphocytes and monocytes and a markedly elevated CSF protein of 1190 mg/l raised the suspicion of an acute encephalitis, since cranial MRI had shown several multifocal acutely demyelinating subcortical lesions. Oligoclonal bands were positive in CSF. Screening for vasculitis and neurotropic viruses including HIV was normal. Transthoracic echocardiography was performed to rule out endocarditis. Neurovascular studies using extracranial and transcranial duplex ultrasound were normal. However, transcranial magnetic stimulation revealed a lesion of the pyramidal tracts to both tibialis anterior muscles.

The patient's condition was interpreted as ADEM, and he was given a 5-day course of high dose intravenous methylprednisolone (500 mg o.d.) which led to a good improvement of the patient's symptoms. He was then discharged into a rehabilitation facility.

Follow-up

Ten weeks later he was referred back from the rehabilitation center, because he had suddenly developed an expressive aphasia and a right-side hemiparesis. On neurological examination, he had additional spastic-ataxic paraparesis, but was still ambulatory. MRI showed a progression of the white matter lesions with a hemorrhagic transformation of a large left temporal lesion. Repeated CSF studies showed pleocytosis with 85–113 cells/mm^3. The further laboratory evaluation did not reveal any specific cause except for a positive polymerase chain reaction for herpes simplex virus in one single CSF examination. Therefore, therapy with i.v. aciclovir was started and continued for 3 weeks without any success. However, his condition further deteriorated during the following 4 weeks, until he was severely aphasic with fluctuating alertness and phases of organic delirium. Cerebral angiography was normal.

Finally, an open meningeal biopsy revealed chronic inflammatory changes in the vessel wall of a small meningeal artery, indicating isolated angiitis of the CNS. The patient was then treated with i.v. cyclophosphamide and high-dose cortico-steroids. This led to a marked improvement of symptoms over the following 4 weeks. The patient was finally discharged with a therapy that consisted of cyclophosphamide (100 mg o.d.) and methylprednisolone (60 mg o.d.) into a rehabilitation facility, still severely dysphasic, but ambulatory with a right sided spastic hemiparesis and a left visual field defect. During a follow-up of 3 years, the patient had no relapse of symptoms.

Image findings

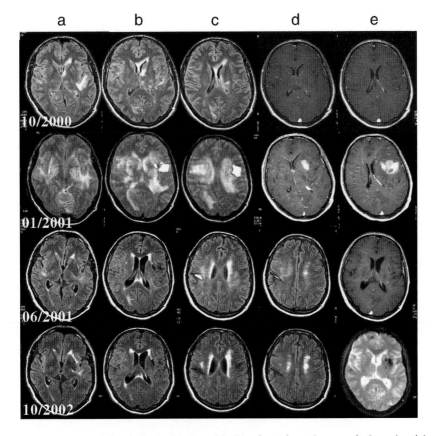

Figure 46.1 10/2000: T$_2$-weighted FLAIR images (a)–(c) show hyperintense lesions involving the corpus callosum, subcortical structures, the thalamus but also left insular and right occipital cortex. T$_1$-weighted contrast enhanced images (d)–(e) show no signs of pathological enhancement. 01/2001: Corresponding to clinical symptoms T$_2$-weighted images show (a)–(e) severe progression of hyperintense lesions now involving bilateral subcortical regions and acute left temporo-parietal hemorrhage. Contrast-enhanced T$_1$-weighted images (d)–(e) show hyperintensity exceeding the bleeding and indicating blood–brain barrier disruption. 06/2001: (a)–(d) After diagnosis was established and adequate treatment administered, extensive hyperintense involvement of the white matter was reversible on T$_2$-weighted images; there was no pathological enhancement on postcontrast images (e). 10/2002: Follow-up examinations showed residual hyperintensity of the white matter on T$_2$-weighted FLAIR (a)–(d) images without signs of progression. T$_2^*$-weighted images show residual blood in the left temporo-parietal region as well as in the right frontal and temporal cortex (e).

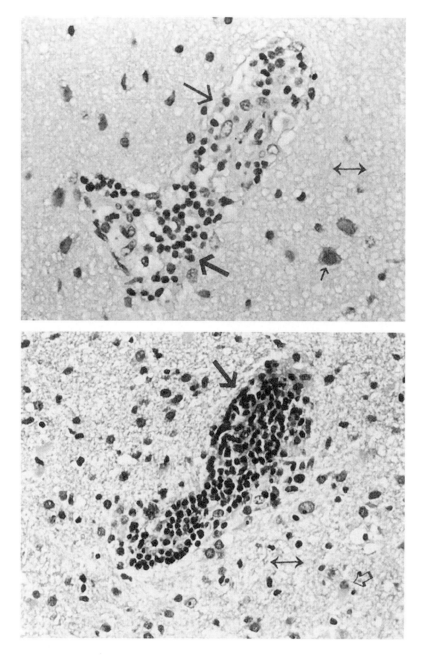

Figure 46.2 Brain biopsy of definite primary angiitis of the CNS (H-E stain). *Upper image*: Indistinct vessel wall with prominent endothelial cells (long thin arrow); lymphocytic inflammation (thick arrow), neuropil edema (double-edged arrow); ischemic necrosis (small arrow). *Bottom image*: Several layers of lymphocytic inflammatory infiltrate (thick arrow); neuropil edema (double arrow); reactive astrocytes (open arrow). Image taken from Alrawi *et al.*, 1999.

Diagnosis

Isolated angiitis of the CNS.

General remarks

The heterogeneous group of inflammatory diseases involving the blood vessels, referred to as vasculitis, can be restricted to the vessels of the central nervous system, without any other apparent systemic lesion, hence termed isolated or primary angiitis or vasculitis of the CNS. A generalized systemic vasculitic process can also involve the CNS, and in such cases, it is referred to as secondary CNS vasculitis. Historically, the disease was called granulomatous angiitis on the basis of granulomata present on postmortem examination, which, however, are not an obligatory feature in histological antemortem studies.

Isolated angiitis of the CNS is an uncommon clinicopathological entity characterized by inflammation of small- and medium-sized vessels. Characteristic mononuclear cell infiltrates of the arterioles are a diagnostic hallmark of the disease; however, vessels of any size may be involved. The initial event causing inflammation of cells is not known. However, the final pathway of inflammation leads to occlusion of the involved blood vessel, thrombosis and, ultimately, ischemia and necrosis of the territories of the involved vessels. Limited data suggest an association with systemic viral illnesses such as cytomegalovirus and varicella-zoster virus, bacteria with strong neuronal tropism or a state of altered host defense (Hodgkin's disease). Besides CSF and serum examinations, MRI, and angiography, the verification of the diagnosis by biopsy is mandatory.

Symptoms and signs are restricted to the nervous system and typically include headaches, encephalopathies and stroke. The new onset of headaches and encephalopathy in association with multifocal signs should provoke diagnostic steps including angiographic and histologic studies.

Special remarks

Immunosuppressive therapy often needs to be maintained for years. In our patient, cyclophosphamide was changed to azathioprine (100 mg o.d., later reduced to 50 mg o.d.) after 12 months, corticoid doses were slowly reduced and finally discontinued after 24 months.

FIRST DESCRIPTION

Hughes, J. T. & Brownell, B. Granulomatous giant-celled angiitis of the central nervous system. *Neurology* 1966; **16**:293–298.

CURRENT REVIEW

Siva, A. Vasculitis of the nervous system. *J. Neurol.* 2001; **248**:451–468.

West, S. G. Central nervous system vasculitis. *Curr. Rheumatol. Rep.* 2003; **5**:116–127.

Younger, D. S. Vasculitis of the nervous system. *Curr. Opin. Neurology* 2004; **17**:317–336.

SUGGESTED READING

Alhalabi, M. & Moore, P. M. Serial angiography in isolated angiitis of the central nervous system. *Neurology* 1994; **44**:1221–1226.

Alrawi, A., Trobe, J. D., Blaivas, M., & Musch, D. C. Brain biopsy in primary angiitis of the central nervous system. *Neurology* 1999; **53**:858–860.

Moore, P. M. & Richardson, B. Neurology of the vasculitides and connective tissue diseases. *J. Neurol. Neurosurg. Psychiatry* 1998; **65**:10–22.

Schmidley, J. *Central Nervous System Angiitis.* Oxford: Butterworth Heinemann, 2000.

Lady who did not want to get up in the morning

Clinical history

A 64-year-old woman seemed quite different to her husband one Sunday morning. She seemed disorganized and was very apathetic. Instead of rising early, preparing breakfast, and heading for work, she seemed content to remain in bed. She denied feeling ill when her husband questioned her. She had a past history of hypertension but was otherwise well.

Examination

She did not volunteer speech. When questioned, there were often long delays in her response. When she did respond, it was very brief and unsustained. She said that she did not feel depressed or sad. Her spoken language and understanding of spoken and written language was normal. Her left face showed minor flattening. Her visual field examination and motor, sensory, and reflexes were normal as was her gait.

BP 160/100. Pulse regular at 80. No heart murmur or neck bruit.

Neurological scores

NIH 0; Barthel Index 100; GCS 15.

Special studies

CT was normal but MRI examination showed a right anterior paramedian thalamic infarct. The infarct was in the territory of the polar (tuberothalamic artery). MRA, ECG, blood, and TEE examinations were all normal.

Image findings

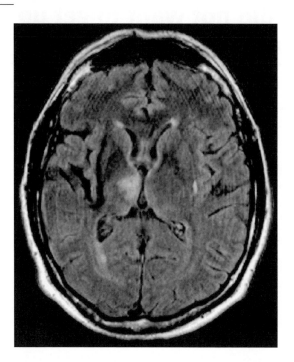

Figure 47.1 MRI examination shows a right paramedian thalamic infarct (T_2-weighted FLAIR image).

Diagnosis

Infarct in the territory of the polar artery.

General remarks

The infarct was in the territory of the polar artery. Figure 47.2(b) shows another polar artery territory infarct on MRI. This vessel has also been variously called the tuberothalamic artery, anterior internal optic artery, and the artery of the premamillary pedicle. The polar artery most often originates from the middle third of the posterior communicating artery. Figures 47.2(a) and 47.2(c) are cartoons that show the location of the various arteries that supply the thalamus. Rarely, the polar artery can arise from the proximal segment of the PCA. There is a great deal of variability of this artery and in about one-third of brains, the polar artery is absent, in which case its territory is supplied by the thalamic–subthalamic

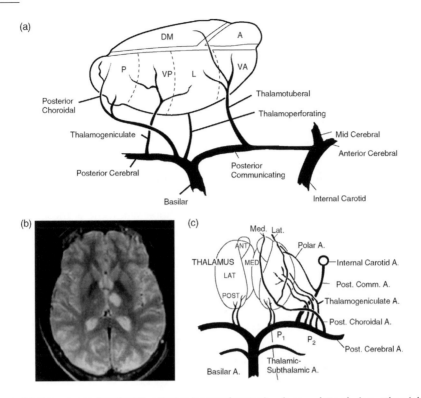

Figure 47.2 (a) A cartoon showing the thalamic supply arteries from a lateral view. The right of the diagram is anterior and the left is posterior. (b) MRI shows a left polar territory thalamic infarct (c) Cartoon showing the thalamic supply arteries from an antero-posterior view.

artery from the same side. The polar artery supplies the anteromedial and ante-rolateral regions of the thalamus but not the anterior nucleus.

In patients with polar artery territory infarcts, motor signs have been minimal or absent. Slight clumsiness or difficulty with rapid alternating movements of the contralateral hand and slight arm drift may be found. Facial asymmetry is common and especially common is the lack of expression in the contralateral side of the face in response to emotional stimuli. Some patients have had minor paresthesias in the contralateral limbs. The major finding has been apathy and abulia. There is usually inertia with decreased spontaneity, decreased amount and volume of speech and decreased spontaneous activity. Answers are usually slow and delayed. Spoken and written replies are terse and tend not to be elaborated on. Patients have difficulty making lists of common things such as fruits, animals, clothing, etc. Patients may also have difficulty organizing pictures temporally. Executive functions such as choice of response, inhibition of a response, choice of actions among alternatives, selection, sequencing and organizing acts and activities, and changing strategies to meet new exigencies, and planning are usually impaired.

Lack of spontaneity is often accompanied by lack of emotional responsivity. The findings of abulia, slowness, lack of insight, and altered executive functions are identical to those found in patients with frontal lobe and caudate nucleus lesions. The dorsomedial nucleus and other thalamic nuclei including VA, VL, and the medial and anterior pulvinar, and anterior nuclear group have strong reciprocal connections with the frontal lobes. The dorsomedial nucleus has strong projections to the anterior cingulate, orbital frontal and dorsolateral frontal cortices. There are a series of parallel thalamo-cortical circuits, which often also involve the caudate nucleus. The frontal lobe syndrome is the most prominent and important finding in patients with polar artery territory infarcts.

SUGGESTED READING

Barth, A., Bogousslavsky, J., & Caplan, L. R. Thalamic infarcts and hemorrhages. In *Stroke Syndromes*, 2nd edn. Cambridge: Cambridge University Press, 2001; 461–468.

Bogousslavsky, J., Regli, J., & Assal, G. The syndrome of tuberothalamic artery territory infarction. *Stroke* 1988; **17**:434–441.

Eslinger, P. J., Warner, G. C., Grattan, L. M., & Easton, J. D. "Frontal lobe" utilization behavior associated with paramedian thalamic infarction. *Neurology* 1991; **41**:450–452.

Graff-Radford, N. R., Eslinger, P. J., Damasio, A. R., & Yamada, T. Non-haemorrhagic infarction of the thalamus: behavioral, anatomic, and physiologic correlates. *Neurology* 1984; **34**:14–23.

Stuss, D. T., Guberman, A., Nelson, R., & La Rochele, S. The neuropsychology of paramedian thalamic infarction. *Brain Cogn.* 1988; **8**:348–378.

Vermont farmer with many spells of rotating and whirling objects

Clinical history

A 77-year-old Vermont farmer had had many spells during the past 3 years. The episodes began abruptly. He senses that things are whirling around. Objects are distorted and often rotated. Sometimes objects are turned upside-down. He often sees double and develops nausea and vomiting and staggers during the attacks. Some attacks are so severe that he falls down. When driving, he sometimes feels that he is turning his truck to the right but, in fact, he is going to the left. In one attack he went across a road. He cannot control his tractor or a car during the attacks. His wife will not drive with him and does not allow the dog to go in his car when he drives. He has chronic hypertension.

Examination

BP 130/80. There is slight right ptosis and horizontal nystagmus on right lateral gaze. The left face is slightly weak. He is deaf in the right ear and has had long-standing tinnitus. He has a slight tremor on finger to nose testing bilaterally. Strength and deep tendon reflexes are normal. The plantar responses are flexor. His gait is wide based and he sometimes lurches to the right.

Neurological scores
NIH 2; Barthel Index 95; GCS 15.

Special studies

CT was normal but MRI examination (Fig. 48.1) showed only white matter hyperintensities and a dilated basilar artery. ECG, blood, and TEE examinations were all normal.

Image findings

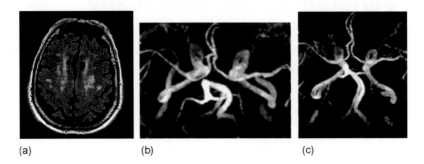

(a)   (b)   (c)

Figure 48.1 (a) MRI, FLAIR ghowing extensive white matter hyperintensities. (b), (c) Intracranial MRA examinations from different angles showing a dilated curved basilar artery.

Diagnosis

Dolichoectatic basilar artery.

General remarks

The episodes that the patient had are best explained by the presence of a dolichoectatic basilar artery. Dolichoectasia describes enlarged, tortuous, and dilated arteries. Since dilatation seems to be the most important feature, the condition is now often referred to as dilatative arteriopathy. Dilatation can be severe in portions of an artery in which case the vessels become fusiform aneurysms. Patients with dolichoectasia also have a higher than expected frequency of penetrating artery disease, the likely cause of the white matter abnormalities shown in Fig. 48.1(a). Knowledge about dilatative arteriopathy is growing but there is still much that is not understood.

Dilatative arteriopathy involves preferentially the intracranial vertebral and basilar arteries. Figures 48.1(b) and 48.1(c) are different views of the dilated tortuous basilar artery. Carotid and middle cerebral artery ectasia occurs but much less often. The clinical findings in patients with intracranial arterial dolichoectasia have now been well described. We know that dilatative arteriopathy can cause strokes. Elongation and angulation of the intracranial arteries can stretch and distort the orifices of arterial branches, leading to decreased blood flow especially in penetrating branches of the large arteries, causing for example basilar artery branch territory infarcts in the pons. Transcranial Doppler studies of dolichoectatic arteries show reduced mean blood flow velocities, with relatively preserved peak flow velocities. Blood flow is often to and fro within the dilated artery causing reduced antegrade flow. Reduced flow can lead to stagnation of the blood column and thrombus formation within the dilated arterial segment. Extensive atherosclerotic plaques – often with calcification, encroachment on the lumen, and thrombus formation – are often found at necropsy. On microscopic examination, there are often fibrotic changes in the vessel wall, with reduced muscularis and attenuated, fragmented, or absent elastica. Luminal thrombi may obstruct arterial branches and portions of the clot can embolize distally. Brain ischemia, either transient or persistent, results. Occasionally, the thin dilated arteries break leading to subarachnoid and brain hemorrhage.

The tortuous elongated arteries can generate pressure and distortion of brain structures especially in the medulla and pons. Stretching of cranial nerves can lead to irritative symptoms such as trigeminal pain and hemifacial spasm and tinnitus. Lower cranial nerve neuropathies are also common.

SUGGESTED READING

Caplan, L. R. Dilatative arteriopathy (Dolichoectasia) *Ann. Neurol.* 2005; **57**:469–471.

DeGeorgia, M., Belden, J., Pao, L., Pessin, M. S., Kwan, E., & Caplan, L. R. Thrombus in vertebrobasilar dolichoectatic artery treated with intravenous urokinase. *Cerebrovasc. Dis.* 1999; **9**:28–33.

Passero, S. & Filosomi, G. Posterior circulation infarcts in patients with vertebrobasilar dolichoectasia. *Stroke* 1998; **29**:653–659.

Pessin, M. S., Chimowitz, M. I., Levine, S. R. *et al.* Stroke in patients with fusiform vertebrobasilar aneurysms. *Neurology* 1989; **39**:16–21.

Pico, F., Labreuche, J., Touboul, P.-J., Leys, D., & Amarenco, P. for the GENIC Investigators. Intracranial arterial dolichoectasia and small vessel disease in stroke patients. *Ann. Neurol.* 2005; **57**:472–479.

Schwartz, A., Rautenberg, W., & Hennerici, M. Dolichoectatic intracranial arteries: review of selected aspects. *Cerebrovasc. Dis.* 1993; **3**:273–279.

Woman with right arm discomfort and sudden blindness

Clinical history

A 45-year-old woman noted right arm discomfort when she began to work around her house. Shortly thereafter, her right eye went blind for a moment and she found that she could not walk. Her husband called 911 and an ambulance took her to an academic medical center near her home.

She had had rheumatic fever as a girl and had been told that she had a murmur. Recently, she had noticed some shortness of breath when she walked quickly or performed difficult housework.

Examination

Her heart rate was 125 and irregular. There was a mitral diastolic murmur with presytolic accentuation. The right hand and arm were cool and white and the fingertips looked grey. There was no radial, ulnar or antecubital arterial pulse.

Vision was now normal in both eyes but she had a left homonymous hemianopia. Cranial nerve examination was otherwise normal except for slight flattening of the left face. The left arm and hand were weak. The right arm was hypotonic and very clumsy on finger-to-nose testing. Deep tendon reflexes were brisker on the left and the left plantar response was extensor. She could not localize touch on her left hand, arm, or face. When she stood, she leaned to the right. Gait was grossly ataxic and she delayed hip flexion on the left.

Neurological scores

NIH 6; Barthel Index 80; GCS 15.

Special studies

MRI examination showed three separate regions of infarction: one in the right cerebral hemisphere in the territory of the right MCA (Fig. 49.1), a second in the left occipital lobe in the territory of the PCA (Fig. 49.2), and an infarct in the right cerebellum in the territory of the right PICA (Fig. 49.3). An aortic arch MRA examination was performed and showed an occlusion of the right innominate artery. Terminal occlusions of branches of the right MCA and PCA were found on intracranial views. An electrocardiogram showed atrial fibrillation and an echocardiogram showed severe mitral stenosis.

Image findings

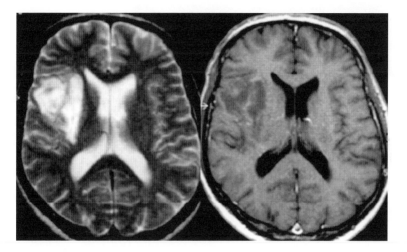

Figure 49.1 T_2 and T_1 weighted MRI scans showing a well-defined infarct in the right cerebral hemisphere.

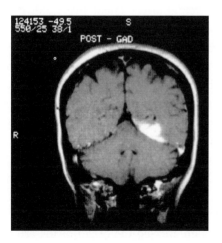

Figure 49.2 T_1 weighted MRI after administration of gadolinium shows hyperintense left occipital lobe infarct with no blood–brain barrier disruption.

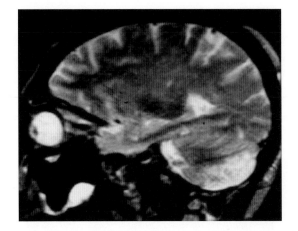

Figure 49.3 Sagittal view of T$_2$-weighted MRI showing an infarct in PICA territory of the cerebellum.

Diagnosis

Innominate artery occlusion due to embolism from mitral stenosis and atrial fibrillation.

General remarks

This patient developed the sudden onset of ischemia of the right upper extremity and nearly simultaneous ischemia in the distribution of branches of the right internal carotid artery (right transient monocular blindness and right MCA territory infarction) and right vertebral artery (right PICA and PCA territory infarction). These findings are diagnostic of innominate artery occlusion, in this case due to embolism from mitral stenosis and atrial fibrillation.

Lesions of the innominate artery are much less common than those of the subclavian arteries and the vertebral arteries. Embolic occlusion of the innominate artery or its branches is more common than intrinsic occlusive disease. Brewster and colleagues reported a large series of 71 patients who had surgery for innominate artery disease during a 20-year period at the Massachusetts General Hospital in Boston. In comparison with subclavian artery and VA disease, in the Massachusetts General Hospital series, there were more varied disease etiologies and patients were, on average, younger and more often women. All patients with atherosclerotic occlusive disease of the innominate artery smoked cigarettes. Atherosclerosis most often affected the origin of the artery from the aortic arch or the proximal third of the vessel.

Takayasu's disease is a common cause of innominate artery occlusion in India, Japan, and in many other countries of the world. Innominate artery aneurysms are often quite large and are of the dissecting or atherosclerotic types. Blunt trauma from motor vehicle accidents, penetrating traumatic injury, and compression of the innominate artery by mediastinal tumors or scar tissue accounted for some instances of innominate artery occlusions.

Occasional patients have had recurrent arm and brain ischemia caused by thrombi within the innominate artery that caused recurrent brain and or eye embolization. In several young patients, no obvious local lesion or coagulopathy was found to explain the floating thrombi but each patient had innominate artery atherosclerotic plaques.

SUGGESTED READING

Brewster, D. C., Moncure, A. C., Darling, C. *et al.* Innominate artery lesions: problems encountered and lessons learned. *J. Vasc. Surg.* 1985; **2**:99–112.

Caplan, L. R. *Posterior Circulation Disease, Clinical Findings, Diagnosis and Management.* Boston: Blackwell Science, 1996.

Ferriere, M., Negre, G., Bellecoste, J. F. *et al.* Thrombus flottant sous-clavier responsable d'un syndrome encephalo-digital, deux observations. *La Presse Med.* 1984; **13**:27–29.

Martin, R., Bogousslavsky, J., Miklossy, J. *et al.* Floating thrombus in the innominate artery as a cause of cerebral infarction in young adults. *Cerebrovasc. Dis.* 1992; **2**:177–181.

A 22-year-old woman with sudden right limb weakness and a mixed aphasia

Clinical history

A 22-year-old caucasian woman was admitted to the emergency room because of sudden right limb weakness and mixed aphasia that she recognized when she woke up.

General history

Normal birth, childhood and adolescence. No infections, no headache.

Examination

On neurological examination, the patient was alert. She had a mixed aphasia and a severe distal right arm and leg sensorimotor paresis.

Neurological scores on admission

NIH 16; Barthel Index 20; GCS 10.

Special studies

Cranial MRI on admission showed an acute large embolic ischemic lesion within the left MCA territory. On intracranial MRA, both MCAs were patent, with the MCA on the left being more accentuated (possibly reflecting hyperperfusion after recanalization). Duplex ultrasound of the extracranial brain supplying arteries revealed pathological flow velocity profiles in both carotid arteries but predominantly on the left. There were concentric hypoechoic lumen obstructions in both CCAs with increasing stenosis in the proximal segments. Flow velocity measures of the VAs revealed slow velocity and slight stenosis at the origin on both sides (left > right). Extracranial MRA showed small calibers of both carotids without circumscribed stenosis.

Ultrasound of the aortic arch and MRI of thoracic and abdominal arteries revealed severe lumen obstructions of the aorta and the large abdominal arteries. Laboratory testing showed slightly increased creatine kinase level 1.4 mmol/l and an elevated erythrocyte sedimentation rate (60 mm at 1 hour). Endovascular aortic biopsy revealed continuous granulomatous inflammation. Lymphocytes and plasma cells with variable numbers of Langhans and foreign-body type giant cells are predominantly localized to the adventitia and outer part of the media.

Image findings

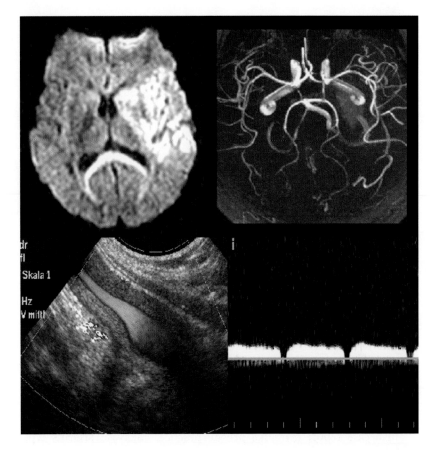

Figure 50.1 *Upper row*: MRI (*left*) and MRA (*right*) on admission, MRI showed left hemispheric DWI lesion indicating acute left MCA stroke. MRA showed patent MCA on both sides. *Bottom row*: Representative images of the Duplex ultrasound examination showing the left CCA (*left*) with massive hypoechoic wall thickening. Flow velocities from the left ICA (*right*) showed pathological flow pattern with systolic deceleration indicating significant proximal vessel obstruction.

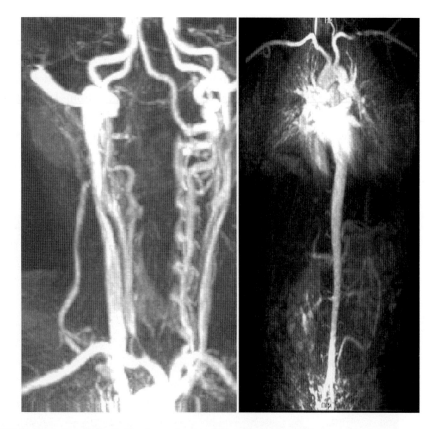

Figure 50.2 Extracranial MRA (*left*) showed very thin diameters of the proximal common carotid arteries. Abdominal MRA (*right*) showed pathological thinning of the aorta and renal arteries.

Diagnosis

Takayasu disease (type 3).

General remarks

In 1830 Rokushu Yamamoto published the first description of Takayasu disease in a case report from his private practice. Takayasu arteritis typically begins between the ages of 15 and 30 years, mostly in Asian and Hispanic populations and is increasingly recognized in Caucasians. The clinical features usually reflect limb or organ ischemia resulting from gradual stenosis of involved arteries, most frequently the thoracic and abdominal aorta and their major branches. Other vessels, such as the pulmonary and coronary arteries, can also be affected. Taking clinical and angiographic findings into account Takayasu arteritis has been classified into the following four types: (1) limited to the aortic arch and its branches; (2) involvement of the thoracic and abdominal aorta and their proximal branches, but sparing the aortic arch; (3) widespread involvement (a combination of types 1 and 2); and (4) involvement of the pulmonary arteries and any of the features of types 1, 2, or 3. This classification has been broadened at the Takayasu Conference in 1994, additionally distinguishing between the presence or absence of coronary (C+/C−) and pulmonary (P+/P−) involvement. Another popular term for the disease was pulseless disease, since radial pulses are often absent or greatly reduced. This is explained by involvement of the subclavian and innominate artery branches of the aortic arch. Takayasu arteritis is a cell-mediated, autoimmune, inflammatory disease. Early and active-stage pathology consists of continuous or patchy granulomatous inflammation, which progresses at variable rates to fibrosis of the intima, media, and adventitia. Cellular infiltrates composed predominantly of lymphocytes and plasma cells are localized to the adventitia and outer part of the media, with variable numbers of Langhans and foreign-body type giant cells (in contrast to giant cell arteritis, in which giant cells tend to lie close to the internal elastic lamina).

Differential diagnosis

Differences between Takayasu arteritis and giant cell arteritis include the following. Takayasu arteritis usually presents prior to the age of 40 years, often involves vascular changes in the upper extremities, with blood pressure differences in the two arms. Giant cell arteritis presents at older ages, is often accompanied by a high sedimentation rate, is often associated with jaw claudication, proximal myalgia, and tenderness along the course of the temporal arteries. With these considerations, Takayasu arteritis can be correctly diagnosed in 90% of cases. Takayasu arteritis targets the large elastic arteries, whereas giant cell arteritis primarily affects the medium-sized muscular arteries with internal and external elastic laminae. Intracranial arteries are almost never involved in giant cell arteritis but represent a major target of the inflammatory response in Takayasu arteritis.

Medical therapy

Steroids and immunosuppressants are usually prescribed empirically. The response rate to monotherapy with steroids is between 20% and 100%. Unresponsive or partially responsive patients may also benefit from immunosuppressants, e.g, methotrexate 10 mg to 25 mg per week (Hoffman, 1995).

Special remarks

In this patient, Takayasu arteritis initially presented with MCA territory stroke in contrast to common initial abdominal or limb symptoms. Moreover, there were almost no typical systemic features as there is hypertension, subclavian steal syndrome, or abdominal or renal abnormalities at the beginning. In this patient initial MRI and cerebrovascular MRA did not lead to the diagnosis, however duplex sonography first showed clear wall thickening with lumen obstruction in the proximal CCA segments leading to diagnosis. Confirmation was achieved by MRA of the aorta and endoscopic biopsy.

CURRENT REVIEW

Numano, F., Okawara, M., Inomata, H., & Kobayashi, Y. Takayasu disease. *Lancet* 2000; **356**:1023–1025.

SUGGESTED READING

Hata, A., Noda, M., Oriwaki, R., & Numano, F. Angiographic findings of Takayasu disease: new classification. *Int. J. Cardiol.* 1996; **54**:155–163.

Hoffman, G. S. Treatment of resistant Takayasu disease. *Rheum. Dis. Clin. North Am.* 1995; **21**:73.

Klos, K., Flemming, K. D., Petty, G. W., & Luthra, H. S. Takayasu's arteritis with arteriographic evidence of intracranial vessel involvement. *Neurology* 2003; **60**:1550–1551.

Michel, B. A., Arend, W. P., & Hunder, G. G. Clinical differentiation between giant cell (temporal) arteritis and Takayasu disease. *J. Rheumatol.* 1996; **23**:106–111.

Weidner, N. Giant-cell vasculitides. *Semin. Diagn. Pathol.* 2001; **18**:24–33.

10-year follow-up of a woman with bilateral MCA disease

Clinical history

We have been regularly following a 56-year-old right-handed woman for 6 years. She presented herself for the first time after she noted a transient left sensory–motor hemiparesis and left homonymous hemianopia caused by a 1/3 right MCA territory stroke.

According to medical records, transcranial Doppler ultrasound and intra-arterial angiography had revealed an occlusion of the M1-segment of the right MCA with good leptomeningeal collateralization, and a low-grade left MCA stenosis. These findings were confirmed during her first presentation in our department. In the meantime, her clinical course had been normal while she was taking clopidogrel.

Examination

Her neurological examination was normal. Her risk factors were slight controlled hypertension and elevated cholesterol and LDL serum levels.

Neurological scores

NIH 0; Barthel Index 100; GCS 15.

Special studies

Extensive diagnostic evaluation including MRI, serial intra-arterial angiography, serum and CSF analysis did not reveal a cause for intracranial arterial disease, e.g., vasculitis or inflammation, coagulation disorders, fibromuscular dysplasia, or Moya Moya syndrome. Family history for cerebrovascular disease was also negative.

MRI at first presentation (Fig. 51.1) showed the T_2-hyperintense chronic lesion in the right parietal MCA territory, congruent with the history of infarction four years ago. MRA showed occlusion of the M1 segment of the right MCA and a proximal stenosis of the left MCA. Correspondingly, there was a delayed contrast bolus arrival on the side of MCA occlusion on PWI (Fig. 51.2A). Consecutive clinical and MRI follow-up visits at regular intervals were performed.

Follow-up

A year later MRA (Fig. 51.2B) showed a progression in the stenosis of the left MCA with significant contrast reduction in the distal portions of the vessel, and a slight beginning hypoperfusion of the left MCA territory on PWI, while the occlusion of the right MCA was persistent.

One year later (Fig. 51.2C), bilateral MCA occlusions and symmetric hypoperfusion of both MCA territories were found. During the period of left MCA stenosis progression, the patient had no cerebrovascular events. All further MRI examinations were unchanged. A recent MRI (Fig. 51.2D) again failed to show any acute or chronic vascular lesions except the old one in the right posterior MCA territory, despite persistent arterial obstruction and hypoperfusion.

Image findings

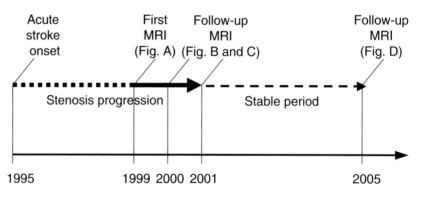

Figure 51.1 (See Fig. 51.2)

Diagnosis

Progressive intracranial arterial obstruction.

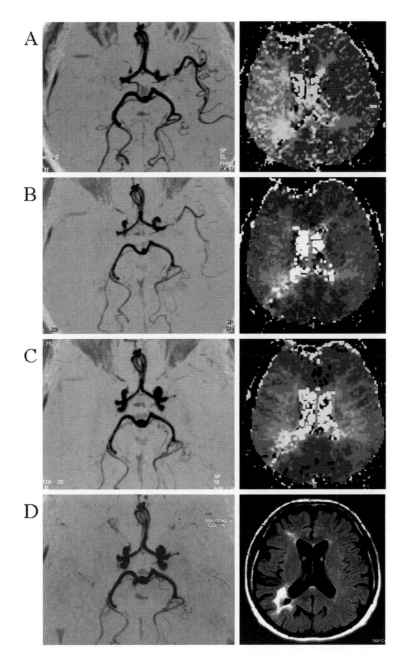

Figure 51.2 MR-Angiography (A–D *left*), perfusion MRI (A–C *right*) and T$_2$-weighted FLAIR image (D *right*) of the patient initially (A) and at follow-up examinations (C–D). For detailed information, see text.

General remarks

This case is unusual because serial MRI and MRA showed progression of an asymptomatic MCA stenosis to occlusion in a patient without ipsilateral cerebral infarction or neurological deficit. This case presentation contrasts to many observations of high recurrence rates of stroke and TIA in patients with progressive MCA stenosis.

Special remarks

MCA occlusions usually reflect signs of embolism without recanalization after prior MCA territory stroke. Asymptomatic MCA occlusions are an uncommon finding in white patients, but more frequent in Asian individuals. Among a series of 18 Japanese patients with asymptomatic MCA occlusion, 4 became symptomatic during a mean observation time of 76 months. According to our own data of 102 patients with MCA disease, the vast majority of patients with MCA occlusion were symptomatic at study entry and were at high-risk for subsequent strokes.

Regarding the pathophysiological concept and brain perfusion studies, the prognosis of patients with MCA occlusion will substantially depend upon the capacity of leptomeningeal collateralization which cannot be visualized non-invasively. This case demonstrates, among few others reported in the literature, that sufficient collateral flow may develop in MCA disease if stenosis progresses gradually over time. However, the exact time that is needed for collaterals to become efficient is unknown, similar to the undetermined influence of other variables like genetic, racial and environmental factors. This lack of systematic data causes the uncertainty on the best therapeutic strategy for these patients: medical treatment like platelet inhibitors or anticoagulation vs. interventional procedures like intracranial angioplasty/stenting vs. extra-intracranial bypass surgery.

SUGGESTED READING

Arenillas, J. F., Molina, C. A., Montaner, J., Abilleira, S., Gonzales-Sanchez, M. A., & Alvarez-Sabin, J. Progression and clinical recurrence of symptomatic middle cerebral artery stenosis: a long-term follow-up transcranial Doppler ultrasound study. *Stroke* 2001; **32**:2898–2904.

Gao, S., Wong, K. S., Hansberg, T., Lam, W. W. M., Droste, D. W., & Ringelstein, E. B. Microembolic signal predicts recurrent cerebral ischemic events in acute stroke patients with middle cerebral artery stenosis. *Stroke* 2004; **35**:2832–2836.

Kern, R., Steinke, W., Daffertshofer, M., Prager, R., & Hennerici, M. Stroke recurrences in symptomatic vs asymptomatic middle cerebral artery disease. *Neurology* 2005; **65**: 859–864.

Miyazawa, N., Hashizume, N., Uchida, M., & Nukui, H. Long-term follow-up of asymptomatic patients with major artery occlusion: rate of symptomatic change and evaluation of cerebral hemodynamics. *Am. J. Neuroradiol.* 2001; **22**:243–247.

Wong, K. S., Gao, S., Chan, Y. L. *et al.* Mechanisms of acute cerebral infarctions in patients with middle cerebral artery stenosis: a diffusion-weighted imaging and microemboli monitoring study. *Ann. Neurol.* 2002; **52**:74–81.

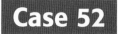

Dysarthria reoccurring after 2 years

Clinical history

A 51-year-old man presented with sudden onset right hemiparesis and dysarthria. Nearly 2 years ago a similar clinical presentation with paresthesia and weakness of the right arm had led to an inpatient assessment at our department. At the time, a megadolicho-basilar artery was diagnosed. A small brainstem stroke was seen on diffusion-weighted MRI and a small hemorrhage into the vessel wall of the basilar artery at the level of infarction was detected. The patient was discharged on warfarin in an attempt to prevent thrombus formation from the irregular vessel wall segment of the basilar artery. Weakness and sensory symptoms subsided during the following 8 weeks.

Examination

Now, 22 months later, the patient presented again with the similar clinical picture of acute onset dysarthria and right hemiparesis. There was additional ataxia, headache and dizziness.

Neurological scores

NIH 6, GCS 15, Barthel 70.

Special studies

MRI showed gross enlargement of the basilar artery to a maximum diameter of 35 mm compressing the pons and mid-brain upwards and leading to gross deformation of pontine tissue. Furthermore, occlusive hydrocephalus was noted with major enlargement of the lateral ventricles and compression of the acqueduct. On ultrasound, both vertebral arteries showed a high resistance flow profile, while the basilar artery had a reduced peak flow velocity. After neurosurgical placement of a ventricular shunt the patient had gradual improvement.

Image findings

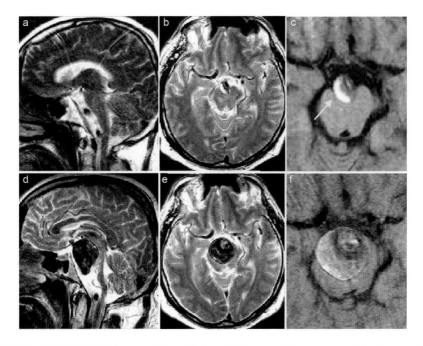

Figure 52.1 (a)–(c) MRI at initial presentation. Note in (c) the small hemorrhage into the vessel wall of an ectactic widened basilar artery. (d)–(f) show follow up MRI scans. The basilar aneurysm had increased from 8 mm to 35 mm in diameter.

Diagnosis

Basilar artery aneurysm growth.

General remarks

Aneurysms of a size larger than 25 mm are commonly called "giant aneurysms." Currently, hemodynamic stress is thought to represent the most likely cause of aneurysms. Hypertension and collagen – vascular diseases are commonly thought of as aggravating conditions, rather than as primary causes of these lesions. Histopathological findings indicate that atherosclerosis may be the essential factor in the pathogenesis of a fusiform aneurysm of the basilar artery in elderly patients. The disrupted internal elastic lamina and muscle layer may be susceptible to mechanical injury by hemodynamic strain, causing progressive attenuation of the arterial wall. Presenting most often with either brainstem compression (including blockage of CSF flow and hydrocephalus) or ischemia, these aneurysms can also rupture.

In a long-term follow-up of 17 patients who were known to have a large or giant aneurysm of the posterior fossa, eight patients received surgical or endovascular treatment for their lesion. The clinical outcome was good recovery in six, moderate disability in one, and vegetative state in one case, respectively. The other nine patients were followed conservatively. Four of them had fatal aneurysmal rupture, and another two patients had worsening of pre-existing symptoms related to their aneurysms. Comparison of the radiographic parameters between those who bled and those who did not bleed showed that those with subsequent rupture had significantly higher rate of aneurysmal thrombus and had a trend for larger diameter of the aneurysm.

Special remarks

This case presents the rapid continuous growth of a giant basilar aneurysm. The MRI shows in much detail the features of giant basilar aneurysms with a residual lumen of normal size and a layered composition of numerous hemorrhages. At least 15 different layers are identified, consisting of a gradually changing characteristic signal arising from different layers of blood. This presentation suggests that, although the follow-up period was short, numerous asymptomatic bleeds must have occurred and show the need for careful monitoring of such patients at stages when more therapeutic options are present. Furthermore, initiation of anticoagulation may in the presence of vessel wall hematoma not only prevent the formation of additional thrombus material, but may also be a predisposing factor to recurrent bleeds.

SUGGESTED READING

Drake, C. G. & Peerless, S. Giant fusiform intracranial aneurysms: review of 120 patients treated surgically from 1965 to 1992. *J. Neurosurg.* 1997; **87**:141–162.

Hassan, T., Ezura, M., & Takahashi, A. Treatment of giant fusiform aneurysms of the basilar trunk with intra-aneurysmal and basilar artery coil embolization. *Surg. Neurol.* 2004; **62**:455–462; discussion 462.

Inamasu, J., Suga, S., Sato, S., Onozuka, S., & Kawase, T. Long-term outcome of 17 cases of large-giant posterior fossa aneurysm. *Clin. Neurol. Neurosurg.* 2000; **102**:65–71.

Nakayama, Y., Tanaka, A., Kumate, S., Tomonaga, M., & Takebayashi, S. Giant fusiform aneurysm of the basilar artery: consideration of its pathogenesis. *Surg. Neurol.* 1999; **51**:140–145.

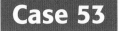

54-year-old man with AVM

Clinical history

A 54-year-old man was witnessed as he had a first ever generalized tonic–clonic seizure. He had no memory of the incident but remembered a strange feeling of coldness and nausea before losing consciousness. He described bilateral occipital headache, but felt well otherwise. His colleagues reported a short moment of disorientation with incoherent speech before he collapsed. In the previous weeks he had been under a lot of stress moving to another city because of a new job.

Medical history revealed osteoporosis, which was treated with risedronate, calcium, and cholecalciferol.

Examination

Neurological examination of the patient was completely normal.

Neurological scores

NIH 0; Barthel Index 100; GCS 15.

Special studies

Non-contrast cranial computed tomography showed a parietooccipital small hyperdense lesion on the right, which was first thought to be a traumatic subarachnoid hemorrhage. However, T_2-weighted MRI sequences revealed a tangle of linear hypointensities consistent with flow-voids in this region. Conventional angiogram confirmed a vascular nidus supplied by enlarged branches of the right middle and posterior cerebral arteries and draining veins to the transverse sinus. Carotid duplex was normal, but transcranial Doppler ultrasonography showed increased flow velocity of the right MCA and the right PCA.

Follow-up

The patient was treated with valproate to prevent recurrence of seizures and had surgical resection of the arteriovenous malformation without complications.

Postoperative angiography showed complete elimination of the arteriovenous malformation.

Image findings

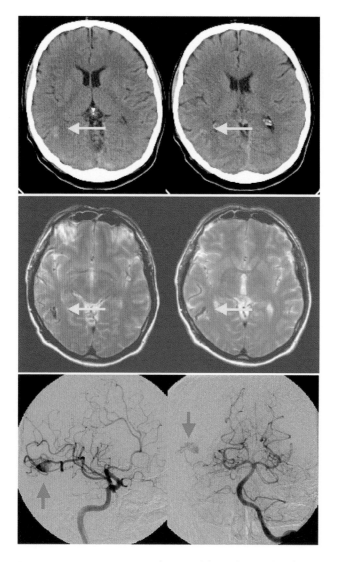

Figure 53.1 *Upper row*: Non-contrast CT shows a right parietooccipital parenchymal hematoma. *Middle row*: T$_2$-weighted axial MRI with corresponding tangle of linear hypointensities consistent with flow-voids. *Bottom row*: Conventional angiogram shows a vascular nidus supplied by enlarged branches of right middle and posterior cerebral arteries.

Diagnosis

Arteriovenous malformation of the brain.

General remarks

Apart from intracranial hemorrage (about 50%) seizures are the most common presentation (about 30%) in patients with arteriovenous malformation of the brain. Seizure types are generalized, focal or focal with generalization in most cases, rarely partial complex or unclassified. Risk factors for seizure presentation in patients with arteriovenous malformation are younger age, male sex, large size, frontal, temporal and parietal location, feeding by a cortical artery or by the middle cerebral artery. The annual risk of hemorrhage is about 2% to 4%. There is a controversy whether or not arteriovenous malformations that have not bled should be treated because of the possible fatal complications of therapy. Treatment options are surgical resection, endovascular treatment, and radiotherapy. While the best-known therapy of arteriovenous malformation is surgical resection, embolization to reduce the vasculature, and radiotherapies are being used increasingly. A trial has just begun to study medical vs. aggressive treatment in patients with AVMs that have not bled.

Special remarks

The Spetzler–Martin scale uses a five-point grading system including size, location, and pattern of venous drainage as characteristics of lesion for the estimation of treatment risks. It classifies patients according to the three elements of *size* (scored 1, small size, for maximum diameter of <3 cm; 2, medium size, for diameter 3 to 6 cm; and 3, large size, for diameter >6 cm), *drainage* (scored 1 for AVM with any drainage into the internal, "deep" cerebral venous system), and *location* (scored 1 for AVM in functionally important brain regions).

This patient was classified as a Spetzler–Martin grade II (small size, location at a non-eloquent site, draining in the transverse sinus).

SUGGESTED READING

Choi, J. H. & Mohr, J. P. Brain arteriovenous malformations in adults. *Lancet Neurol.* 2005; **4**:299–308.

Spetzler, R. F. & Martin, N. A. A proposed grading system for arteriovenous malformations. *Neurosurgery* 1986; **65**:476–483.

The Arteriovenous Malformation Study Group. Arteriovenous malformations of the brain in adults. *N. Engl. J. Med.* 1999; **340**:1812–1818.

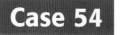

Alternating transient numbness

Clinical history

A 59-year-old woman noticed transient loss of feeling in her right arm and leg. She reported similar symptoms twice during the past week, however, also affecting the left trunk and the entire left side of the body. She also described an unsteadiness of gait.

The patient had no history of cerebrovascular disease. As a heavy smoker (40 pack–years) she had chronic bronchitis. There were no clinical symptoms of an infection.

She had hypertension for 10 years, treated with bisoprolol and ramipiril, and hyperlipoproteinemia treated with simvastatin.

Examination

Neurological examination showed a slight proximal motor deficit of the left arm with increased tendon reflexes. Babinski sign was positive bilaterally. Her gait was unsteady. Her legs were strong and sensation tests were normal.

Neurological scores

NIH 1; Barthel Index 90; GCS 15.

Special studies

MRI scan showed bihemispheric acute ischemic lesions on diffusion-weighted imaging, while perfusion MRI showed a delayed contrast agent bolus arrival time in both MCA territories compared to the posterior territory. Bilateral proximal stenosis of the ICA was seen on MRA and confirmed by duplex sonography. Intracranial collateral flow from the basilar system was observed using transcranial Doppler duplexsonography.

Extensive evaluation including transesophageal echocardiography showed normal atrial and ventricular sizes without intracavitary thrombi, and normal valves. There were no septal defects or a patent foramen ovale. There was no evidence for pathological valves suggestive of endocarditis. No relevant atherosclerosis of the aortic arch was found. Routine laboratory testing showed elevated CRP (10.3 mg/l), without elevated white blood count or other pathological findings. Urinalysis detected urinary tract infection with elevated leukocytes, further microbiological testing showed infection with *Escherichia coli*. Routine and advanced coagulation studies showed only an elevated D-dimer, consistent with cerebral ischemia, other parameters especially fibrinogen were normal. Other serological analyses showed no systemic infection; no antibodies against *Chlamydia pneumoniae* were found.

Follow-up

As no other causes of a possible source of embolism were found, the patient was diagnosed with synchronic symptomatic bilateral ICA stenosis and treated with consecutive thrombendarterectomy. After thrombendarterectomy of the right side, the right ICA showed normal flow, now with intracranial cross flow from the right to the left side via the anterior communicating artery in TCD. This collateralization pattern normalized after subsequent thrombendarterectomy of the left ICA.

Image findings

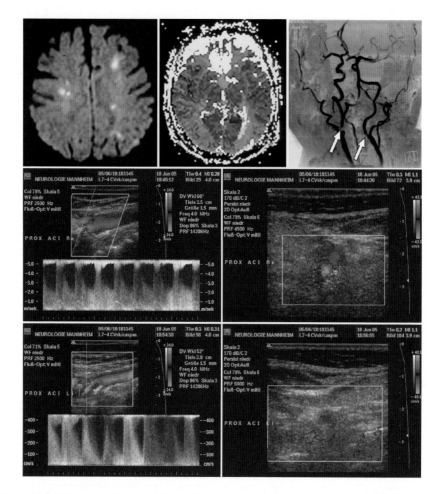

Figure 54.1 Initial MRI scan, showing bihemispheric acute ischemic lesions on diffusion weighted imaging (DWI, *left*). Perfusion-weighted imaging (PWI, *middle*) shows delayed contrast agent bolus arrival in both MCA territories compared to the PCA territories. TOF MRA (right) shows bilateral proximal ICA stenoses. Duplex ultrasound of the right ICA (middle row) and left ICA (bottom row) in the axial (left) and transverse plane (right): Stenosis of the right ICA with lumen reduction of 85% and peak systolic flow velocity of more than 500 cm/s, and stenosis of the left ICA with 70% lumen reduction and peak systolic flow velocity of more than 400 cm/s.

Diagnosis

Synchronic bihemispheric stroke due to bilateral carotid artery stenosis.

General remarks

Multiple brain infarcts are highly suggestive of a proximal source of embolism, especially of a cardiac origin. It was found that acute bilateral stroke in the anterior circulation was associated with embolism arising from the heart in 25%. A cardiac source etiology was described of multiple brain infarcts in 31%. In another recent study, 95 out of 329 consecutive patients were identified as having acute multiple brain infarcts using diffusion-weighted MRI. The authors found that, in strokes affecting both the anterior and the posterior circulation, cardioembolism was the most frequent cause (6 out of 11 patients). However, if the anterior circulation was affected bilaterally, large artery atherosclerosis was the most common etiology (9 out of 20 patients). In this patient the multiple stereotyped attacks in the same vascular territory indicated local hypoperfusion in the right carotid territory making it likely that the acute process involved the right ICA or its branches.

ICA disease can also result in PCA territory strokes in those patients in which PCA originates from the ICA (fetal type PCA). Stroke patterns may give clues to stroke mechanism; however, thorough evaluation using transcranial duplex ultrasound, MR angiography and cardiac investigations (Holter ECG, echocardiography) are needed.

Trigger factors of synchronic acute symptomatic bilateral extracranial stenosis might be systemic infections, or inflammatory disease, although reliable data for this correlation are still missing. The high CRP level (perhaps related to smoking) might explain the activity of her carotid artery plaques.

Treatment options in carotid stenosis are surgical (thrombendarterectomy) or interventional (stenting). In the particular case of bilateral carotid stenosis, an individualized approach according to the risk profile of the patient and the experience of the surgeon/interventionalist is crucial. A general recommendation could currently not be given; this point is subject of diverse ongoing trials (e.g., the SPACE trial).

Special remarks

In this case, we ruled out other possible causes of cardioembolism, substantiating the diagnosis of bilateral symptomatic ICA stensosis.

Bihemispheric ischemic lesions due to simultaneous embolism from both ICAs in patients with bilateral ICA stenosis is an uncommon finding. Agents triggering the plaque rupture have to be assumed. Possible factors increasing the vulnerability of the plaques seem to degrade the plaque matrix. A crucial key point is the activation of matrix metalloproteinases. There is common agreement about several infectious conditions initiating this process. Our patient only had a urinary tract infection with *E. coli*. Whether this was a possible mechanism is speculative.

FIRST DESCRIPTION

Clark, E. & Harrison, C. V. Bilateral carotid artery obstruction. *Neurology* 1956; **6**:705–715.

SUGGESTED READING

Bogousslavsky, J., Bernasconi, A., & Kumral, E. Acute multiple infarction involving the anterior circulation. *Arch. Neurol.* 1996; **53**:50–57.

Hennerici, M. G. The unstable plaque. *Cerebrovasc. Dis.* 2004; **17**:17–22.

Lindsberg, P. J. & Grau, A. J. Inflammation and infections as risk factors for ischemic stroke. *Stroke* 2003; **34**:2518–2532.

Reinhard, M., Muller, T., Roth, M., Guschlbauer, B., Timmer, J., & Hetzel, A. Bilateral severe carotid artery stenosis or occlusion – cerebral autoregulation dynamics and collateral flow patterns. *Acta Neurochir.* (Wien) 2003; **145**:1053–1059.

Ringleb, P. A., Allenberg, J., Hennerici, M. *et al.* On behalf of the SPACE Collaboration Group. 30 day results from the SPACE trial of stent-protected angioplasty versus carotid endarterectomy in symptomatic patients: a randomised trial. *Lancet* 2006; **368**:1–8.

Roh, J. K., Kang, D. W., Lee, S. H., Yoon, B. W., & Chang, K. H. Significance of acute multiple brain infarction on diffusion-weighted imaging. *Stroke* 2000; **31**:688–694.

Rothwell, P. M., Metha, Z., Howard, S. C., Gutnikov, S. A., & Warlow, C. P. Treating individuals 3: from subgroups to individuals: general principles and the example of carotid endarterectomy. *Lancet* 2005; **365**:256–265.

Sloan, M. A. & Haley, E. C. Jr. The syndrome of bilateral hemispheric border zone ischemia. *Stroke* 1990; **21**:1668–1673.

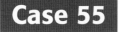

Typical intracerebral hemorrhage – or not?

Clinical history

A 57-year-old man reported the sudden onset of right-side headache and weakness of his left limbs. Except for smoking (about 35 pack–years), and regular but moderate alcohol drinking, there were no cerebrovascular risk factors or diseases in the patient's medical history.

Examination

Neurological examination showed a slightly drowsy patient with severe sensorimotor hemiparesis on the left with positive Babinski sign. Blood pressure at admission was normal and there were no signs of traumatic injury.

Neurological scores

NIH 11; Barthel Index 45; GCS 14.

Special studies

Non-contrast CT showed intracerebral hematoma in the right thalamus with intraventricular extension and only minimal if any surrounding edema. An MRI was performed 48 hours later. Axial T_2^*-susceptibility-weighted – blood sensitive - images showed hypointense correlate of hemorrhage in the right thalamus, now with surrounding vasogenic edema, that was hyperintense on T_2^* scans, as well as diffusion-weighted images, and mass effect on the right lateral ventricle. In addition, however diffusion-weighted images revealed a tiny acute ischemic lesion in the occipital pole of the right PCA territory. On MRA, both PCAs showed signal loss in the proximal P2-segment. Bilateral PCA stenosis was confirmed by transcranial Doppler ultrasound.

Facilitated by MRI findings, the diagnosis of a secondary hemorrhagic transformation of thalamic stroke with an additional occipital acute ischemic lesion and bilateral P2 stenosis was made.

Image findings

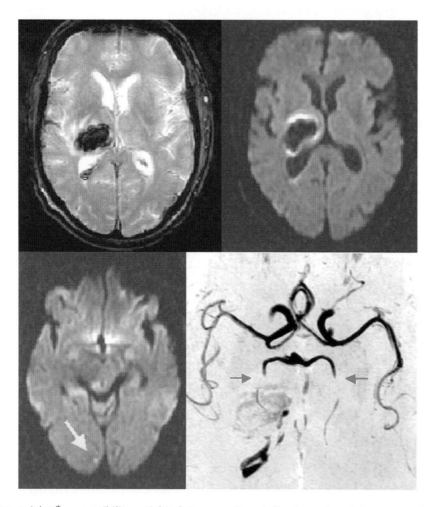

Figure 55.1 Axial T_2^*-susceptibility-weighted images (*top left*) show hypointense correlate of hemorrhage in the right thalamus with surrounding vasogenic edema, which is hyperintense in T_2^* as well as on diffusion-weighted images (*top right*). Additional low signal indicating blood in the posterior horn of the lateral ventricle is seen. Diffusion-weighted image show additional tiny acute ischemic lesion in the occipital pole of the right PCA territory (*bottom left*, arrow). On MRA both PCAs show signal loss in the proximal P2-segment (*bottom right*, arrow).

Diagnosis

Secondary hemorrhagic transformation of thalamic infarct.

General remarks

The most common cause of intracerebral hemorrhages (55%–65%) is arterial hypertension. Acute hypertension leads to sudden arterial stress and rupture of previously normal arterioles and capillaries. Chronic, poorly controlled arterial hypertension leads to degenerative processes within the arterial wall affecting predominantly the perforating arteries of basal ganglia and brainstem. In case of a sudden increase of blood pressure (e.g., patient coughs), these vessels can easily rupture. Hemorrhages in this location are often called "typical" in contrast to lobar hemorrhages, the so-called "atypical" ones (e.g., in patients with CAA).

Although prospective studies are not available up to date, it is estimated that 1%–6% of ischemic strokes show secondary hemorrhagic transformation or parenchymal bleeding.

Vascular congestion of varying degree is common to all ischemic strokes, but extravasation of blood is often associated with embolic infarcts, because emboli tend to migrate and lyse, and recirculate into the infarcted brain. This type of hemorrhagic transformation occurs 12 h to 36 h after stroke onset and is most often asymptomatic. This type of secondary hemorrhagic transformation must be distinguished from primary hemorrhage into mostly large infarcts that is almost always accompanied by clinical worsening. In addition, the underlying pathology (e.g. NVAF) needs to be identified for secondary prevention measures. In their absence as in this case, the etiology of the PCA disease is uncertain, but dissections do involve this vessel and can explain the unusual hemorrhage.

Special remarks

This case emphasizes the need for a complete evaluation of all possible aetiologies of stroke, even if at first sight everything seems to be obvious. If there had been no magnetic resonance imaging, according to the cranial CT and the bleeding location, this case could have been taken as a "typical" intracerebral hemorrhage. This case supports the possibility that some cases of apparently primary intracerebral hemorrhages might be due to secondary hemorrhagic transformation of infarct.

SUGGESTED READING

Berger, C., Fiorelli, M., Steiner, T. *et al.* Hemorrhagic transformation of ischemic brain tissue: asymptomatic or symptomatic? *Stroke* 2001; **32**:1330–1335.

Bogousslavsky, J., Regli, F., Uske, A., & Maeder, P. Early spontaneous hematoma in cerebral infarct: is primary cerebral hemorrhage overdiagnosed? *Neurology.* 1991; **41**:837–840.

Caplan, L. R., Estol, C. J., & Massaro, A. R. Dissection of the posterior cerebral arteries *Arch. Neurol.* 2005; **62**:1138–1143.

Mead, G. E., Wardlaw, J. M., Dennis, M. S., & Lewis, S. C. Extensive haemorrhagic transformation of infarct: might it be an important cause of primary intracerebral haemorrhage? *Age Ageing* 2002; **31**:429–433.

Tong, D. C., Adami, A., Moseley, M. E., & Marks, M. P. Prediction of hemorrhagic transformation following acute stroke: role of diffusion- and perfusion-weighted magnetic resonance imaging *Arch. Neurol.* 2001; **58**:587–593.

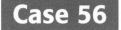

The butcher and his wife

Clinical history

A 74-year-old woman was referred to Neurology because of sudden difficulty in walking and cognitive changes. Despite her age, she still worked behind the counter in her family's butcher's shop. According to her husband she had been well until 1 year earlier, when she began to fall occasionally. However, until now, this and memory lapses once in a while had not interfered with her work or daily living.

Examination

On neurological examination she had an unsteady, wide-based gait, pyramidal tract signs on the right and reduced sensation of vibration and proprioception below the knees. Muscle strength and tone were normal. She achieved 22 of 30 points in the Mini-Mental State Examination. She was emotionally labile with sudden short episodes of crying or laughing during the examination. She was not able to provide a detailed account of her daily routines.

Neurological scores
NIH 4; Barthel Index 70; GCS 15.

Special studies

On MRI, T_2-weighted sequences showed areas of increased signal intensity in the periventricular, subcortical, and pontine white matter. In addition, an acute, hyperintense lesion on DWI was found in the splenium of the corpus callosum.

Follow-up

During the next 4 weeks, the falls and memory lapses became more prominent until she became bedridden, incontinent, and completely dependent. MRI revealed multiple small acute ischemic lesions on DWI. Finally, she had to be cared for in a nursing home.

Image findings

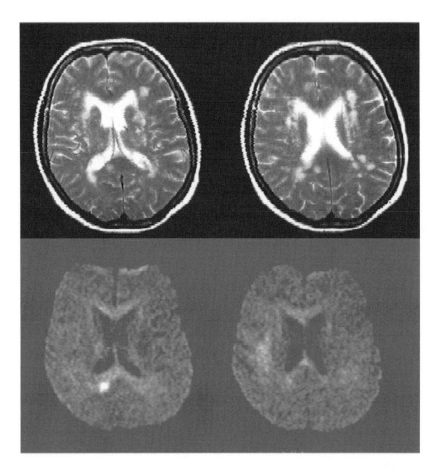

Figure 56.1 T$_2$-weighted images (upper row) show distinct hyperintense changes in the periventricular white matter. DWI (bottom row) identifies an acute ischemic lesion in the right splenium of the corpus callosum.

Diagnosis

Progressive SVE.

General remarks

SVE or leukoaraiosis – from the Greek roots *leuko* (white) and *araiosis* (rarified) – is characterized by patchy or diffuse abnormalities in the deep white matter, which appear as low attenuation on CT or high intensity signal on T_2-weighted MRI sequences. These abnormalities are seen characteristically in the periventricular regions, especially around the horns of the lateral ventricles, in the centrum semiovale and in the brainstem. These findings should be distinguished from incidental, similar but less severe changes unrelated to clinical manifestations, which may be seen in the elderly population. On the other hand, microangiopathic lesions are also found in up to 70% of persons with vascular dementia and Alzheimer's disease and can occur in a large variety of clinical entities.

The clinical features of SVE include a reduction in the amount of activity and speech, latencies in responding to queries and conversation, and short terse responses. Executive functions are reduced and the findings include dementia, incontinence, small-stepped gait, changes in speed, affect, emotional lability, as well as memory deficits. Neurological signs found are dysarthria, pseudobulbar palsy, grasp reflex, pyramidal signs, paraplegia in flexion, and akinetic mutism. These symptoms are believed to be caused by interruption of prefrontal subcortical circuits. These circuits are known to be involved in the executive control of working memory, organization, language, mood, regulation of attention, constructional skills, motivation, and socially responsive behaviors.

Special remarks

As cognitive impairment with executive dysfunction may be clinically silent in the early phase of disease, a thorough neurological and psychiatric examination of these patients, the evaluation of gait and falls, timed-walk, timed finger-tapping, and frontal bladder control (urge incontinence and nocturia) are important to determine the functional status and disability. Relatives and caregivers may report behavioral changes.

In the presence of chronic microangiopathy or previous stroke, an acute ischemic lesion can lead to an aggravation of neurological deficits, with predominant disturbances of either vigilance or cognitive functions. The clinical characteristics of such syndromes may not necessarily be dominated by the new lesion. In particular, patients with chronic tissue changes are at risk to develop severe clinical syndromes, despite the occurrence of only small acute lesions. This indicates the existence of a well-balanced network, compensating for subclinical structure damage.

Differential diagnosis and management

A similar clinical picture can occasionally develop in patients with intravascular lymphoma. In that case there are also often skin lesions and a rapidly deteriorating course. Occasionally, patients with amyloid angiopathy, especially with coexistent granulomatous angiitis can present similar clinical and imaging findings. In patients with SVE whole blood viscosity may be important in explaining new infarcts. Flow through narrowed small arteries and capillaries is influenced greatly by the viscosity of the fluid that goes through these channels. The hematocrit and fibrinogen levels are the two most important components of viscosity. Some patients have relatively high hematocrits because they do not drink adequate fluids. Attention to blood pressure, hematocrit, fibrinogen levels, and fluid intake is useful in attempting to prevent further brain damage in patients with SVE.

SUGGESTED READING

Beal, M. F. & Fisher, C. M. Neoplastic angioendotheliosis. *J. Neurol. Sci.* 1982; **53**:359–375.

Caplan, L. R. Binswanger's disease-revisited. *Neurology* 1995; **45**:626–633.

Caplan, L. R. & Schoene, W. C. Clinical features of subcortical arteriosclerotic encephalopathy (Binswanger disease). *Neurology* 1978; **28**:1206–1215.

Ernst, E. & Resch, K. L. Fibrinogen as a cardiovascular risk factor: a meta-analysis and review of the literature. *Ann. Intern. Med.* 1993; **118**:956–963.

Fisher, C. M. Binswanger's encephalopathy: a review. *J. Neurol.* 1989; **236**:65–79.

Gootjes, L., Teipel, S. J., & Zebuhr, Y. Regional distribution of white matter hyperintensities in vascular dementia, Alzheimer's disease and healthy aging. *Dement. Geriatr. Cogn. Disord.* 2004; **18**:180–188.

Greenberg, S. M., Vonsattel, J. P. G., Stakes, J. W., Gruber, M., & Finkelstein, S. P. The clinical spectrum of cerebral amyloid angiopathy: presentations without lobar hemorrhage. *Neurology* 1993; **43**:2073–2079.

Grotta, J., Ackerman, R., Correia, J. *et al.* Whole blood viscosity parameters and cerebral blood flow. *Stroke* 1982; **13**:296–301.

Ishii, N., Nishihara, Y., & Imamura, T. Why do frontal lobe symptoms predominate in vascular dementia with lacunes? *Neurology,* 1986; **36**:340–345.

Kaste, M. & Erkinjuntti, T. MRI correlates of executive dysfunction in patients with ischaemic stroke. *Eur. J. Neurol.* 2003; **10**:625–631.

Mezzapesa, D. M., Rocca, M. A., Pagani, E., Comi, G., & Filippi, M. Evidence of subtle gray-matter pathologic changes in healthy elderly individuals with nonspecific white-matter hyperintensities. *Arch. Neurol.* 2003; **60**:1109–1112.

Olszewski, J. Subcortical arteriosclerotic encephalopathy. *World Neurol.* 1965; **3**:359–374.

Pantoni, L., Poggesi, A., Basile, A. M. *et al.* On behalf of the LADIS Study Group. Leukoaraiosis predicts hidden global functioning impairment in nondisabled older people: The LADIS (Leukoaraiosis and Disability in the Elderly) Study. *J. Am. Geriatr. Soc.* 2006; **54**:1095–1101.

Rockwood, K., Burns, A., Gauthier, S., & DeKosky, S. T. Vascular cognitive impairment. *Lancet Neurol.* 2003; **2**:89–98.

Schmidt, R., Enzinger, C., Ropele, S., Schmidt, H., & Fazekas, F. Austrian Stroke Prevention Study. Progression of cerebral white matter lesions: 6-year results of the Austrian Stroke Prevention Study. *Lancet* 2003; **361**:2046–2048.

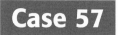

Malignant MCA infarction

Clinical history

A 32-year-old woman was found by her daughter lying in bed in the morning, seemingly asleep. Because she was unable to awaken her mother, the girl called an ambulance. Paramedics reported the woman was comatose and had a right-sided hemiparesis.

Examination

The patient was comatose, but showed fluctuating vigilance. Pupils were normal. She did not speak or follow instructions. There was no response to painful stimuli to the right extremities. Babinski's sign was positive on the right.

Neurological scores

NIH 19; Barthel Index 0; GCS 8.

Special studies

CT scan showed hypodensity in two-thirds of the left MCA territory, consistent with a large hemispheric infarction. At this point, there was already slight midline shift, as well as trapping of the left lateral ventricle. Ultrasound revealed a distal occlusion of the left internal carotid artery, next to an occlusion of the left middle cerebral artery.

Course and treatment

In the following 3 hours the patient developed a dilated pupil on the left and became less responsive to painful stimuli. Surgical decompression was performed.

Follow-up

There were no postoperative complications. The ICA and MCA showed complete recanalization. Extensive evaluation did not find a source of embolism – dissection of the ICA was considered as a possible pathomechanism of stroke. Over the course of the next 2 weeks, the patient remained awake, had a global aphasia, showing slight comprehension, and a high grade hemiparesis on the right. She was thereafter transferred to a rehabilitation clinic.

Image findings

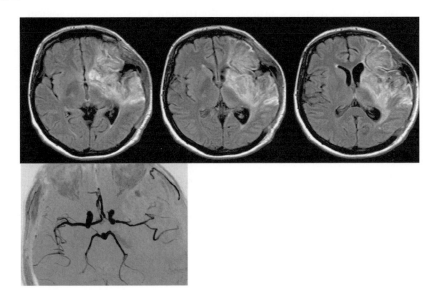

Figure 57.1 Postoperative MRI performed 1 week after hemicraniectomy. *Upper row:* T$_2$-weighted FLAIR images show a hyperintense lesion in the left hemisphere affecting approximately two-thirds of the MCA territory. Note residual bulging of brain tissue to the left, but no compression of the ventricles or midline structures. *Bottom row:* Initially occluded MCA and ICA have recanalized.

Diagnosis

Space-occupying left MCA stroke and subsequent hemicraniectomy.

General remarks

Brain edema in patients with acute stroke occurs during the first hours after infarction, peaks on the second or third day, but can cause mass effect for up to 10 days. Between 5% and 10% of patients develop enough cerebral edema to cause obtundation or brain herniation. Brainstem compression may result in coma and respiratory arrest.

Osmotherapy is recommended for patients whose condition is deteriorating secondary to increased intracranial pressure, including those with herniation syndromes. Water restriction and intravenous mannitol may be used to raise the serum osmolarity, but hypovolemia should be avoided as this can contribute to hypotension and worsen infarction (4×250 ml of 10% glycerol over 30–60 minutes i.v., or 25–50 g mannitol every 3 to 6 hours i.v.).

Surgical decompression and evacuation of a large hemispheric infarction are life-saving. Survivors, however, often retain a residual neurological deficit. In a recent prospective small case series, surgical decompressive therapy in hemispheric space-occupying infarction lowered mortality from 80% to 30% without increasing the rate of severely disabled survivors. Early decompressive surgery, within the first 24 hours after stroke onset, can reduce mortality even more markedly.

Special remarks

The laterality of the infarction is reported not to have a prognostic relevance. However, there might be a tendency for physicians not to consider surgery to patients with left-sided strokes, as subsequent neurological deficit is judged to be more severely disabling in the dominant hemisphere. This patient strengthens that the timing of surgery is of greater importance than the laterality of the lesion.

SUGGESTED READING

Erban, P., Woertgen, C., Luerding, R., Bogdahn, U., Schlachetzki, F., & Horn, M. Long-term outcome after hemicraniectomy for space occupying right hemispheric MCA infarction. *Clin. Neurol. Neurosurg.* 2005 Aug 29.

Schwab, S., Steiner, T., Aschoff, A. *et al.* Early hemicraniectomy in patients with complete middle cerebral artery infarction. *Stroke* 1998; **29**:1888–1893.

Serena, J., Blanco, M., Castellanos, M. *et al.* The prediction of malignant cerebral infarction by molecular brain barrier disruption markers. *Stroke* 2005; **36**:1921–1926.

The DESTINY Study Group. DESTINY-Decompressive Surgery for the treatment of malignant Infarction of the MCA – preliminary results. *Cerebrovasc. Dis.* 2006; **27**:59.

Thomalla, G. J., Kucinski, T., Schoder, V. *et al.* Prediction of malignant middle cerebral artery infarction by early perfusion- and diffusion-weighted magnetic resonance imaging. *Stroke* 2003; **34**:1892–1899.

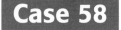

Stroke in Recklinghausen's disease

Clinical history

A 44-year-old woman developed transient weakness of the right arm and leg lasting for about 30 minutes. There were no known vascular risk factors. However, the patient was known to have sporadic Recklinghausen's disease. She had been operated on for a 3×2 cm angioectatic retroauricular neurofibroma on the left 2 years ago.

Examination

On admission, the patient was alert and showed no focal neurological signs. She had several subcutaneous tumors that were known from previous examinations and were already identified as neurofibromas.

Neurological scores
NIH 0; Barthel Index 100; GCS 15.

Special studies

Initial CT scan in the emergency unit was normal. During ultrasound examination the next day the patient suddenly developed moderate paresis of the right arm and slight mixed aphasia. Ultrasound and MRA showed a large carotid aneurysm in the neck with hypoechoic intraluminal surface structures. During examination, small particles broke away from the surface structures and moved intracranially. This phenomenon preceded the development of the above mentioned acute symptoms. Intravenous thombolysis was administered 11 min after symptom onset without additional brain imaging (since initial CT the day before was normal). Despite the very short time window, there was almost no improvement of function, neurological findings and scores. MRI 2 hours after thrombolysis revealed large DWI hyperintense changes indicating acute stroke.

Neurological scores
NIH 5; Barthel Index 60; Rankin 3.

Follow-up

Surgical resection of the carotid aneurysm on the left was performed 2 weeks after stroke. Histology revealed infiltration of the vessel wall by neurofibromatous tumor mass.

Two weeks after carotid surgery – before discharge – the patient developed acute abdominal symptoms due to an aneurysm of the mesenterial artery and the infrarenal aorta. Four weeks after resection of the mesenterical aneurysm and stenting of the aortic aneurysm, a new aneurysm of the proximal mesenteric artery became symptomatic and had to be surgically removed. The patient was discharged after 4 months. Until then she had recovered from her neurological deficits but still was dependent in daily life activities (Rankin 3).

Neurological scores on discharge

NIH 6; Barthel Index 70; GCS 15.

Image findings

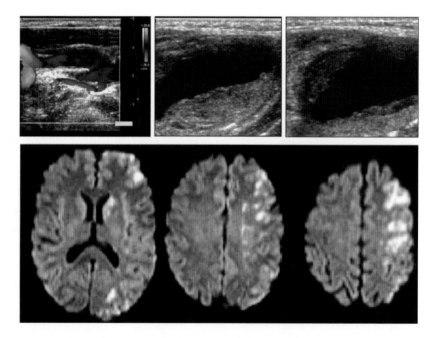

Figure 58.1 Ultrasound images show a large carotid aneurysm with hypoechoic intraluminal surface structures (*upper row*). Diffusion-weighted MRI (*bottom row*) shows multiple acute ischemic lesions in the left anterior and middle cerebral artery territory.

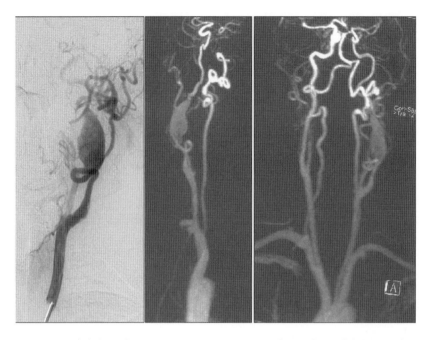

Figure 58.2 Conventional (*left*) and magnetic resonance angiography (*right*) with left carotid aneurysm.

Diagnosis

Carotid aneurysm associated with Recklinghausen's disease with intraluminal neurofibromatous tumor mass.

General remarks

The earliest convincing medical descriptions of what we now know to be neurofibromatosis type 1 occurred in the eighteenth century. However, Friedrich von Recklinghausen put the disorder in the medical lexicon with his correct identification in 1882 of the neural origin of its most common lesion, the neurofibroma. Following this important work, the disorder became known as von Recklinghausen disease. Neurofibromatosis type 1 is the most common form of neurofibromatosis; the 1988 National Institutes of Health Consensus Panel concluded that it was one of the two forms of neurofibromatosis that could be precisely classified at that time. Café au lait spots, peripheral neurofibromas, and Lisch nodules are the clinical manifestations of neurofibromatosis type 1 (Table 58.1).

Stroke as a consequence of Recklinghausen's disease is a very rare condition. Anecdotal cases of smooth intrinsic stenosis or occlusion of major cerebral vessels, most frequently the supraclinoid ICA, or proximal anterior or middle

Table 58.1. Diagnosis of neurofibromatosis type 1

- Six or more café au lait macules over 5mm in greatest diameter in prepubertal individuals and over 15mm in greatest diameter in postpubertal individuals
- Two or more neurofibromas of any type or one plexiform neurofibroma
- Freckling in the axillary or inguinal regions
- Optic glioma
- Two or more Lisch nodules (iris hamartomas)
- A distinctive osseous lesion such as sphenoid dysplasia or thinning of long-bone cortex with or without pseudoarthrosis
- A first-degree relative (parent, sibling, or offspring) with neurofibromatosis type 1 by the above criteria.

cerebral arteries in association with Moyamoya type collateralization, have been reported in neurofibromatosis type 1, but the true incidence is unknown. These patients presented with stroke in childhood. An increased prevalence of stroke from presumed athero-thrombotic cerebrovascular disease has been reported as well. However, this must be interpreted cautiously, because hypertension, for which neurofibromatosis type 1 patients are at increased risk, accounts for some cases and the Moyamoya constriction may be responsible for others. Ten cases of cerebral aneurysms and subarachnoid hemorrhage have been reported. Four had internal carotid constriction, and bleedings may have been related to blood vessel abnormalities rather than to berry aneurysms.

Special remarks

Although a rare condition, vascular complications are well known in Recklinghausen's disease. Aneurysms, however, are most commonly observed at the visceral arteries. This case primarily became symptomatic from carotid aneurysm. Moreover, after initial TIA there was embolization during ultrasound examination that led to immediate thrombolysis (an extremely rare event suggested to occur only once per 100000 examinations). Despite a very short time window there was no beneficial effect of thrombolysis likely due to the fact that the emboli were tumor material rather than thrombi.

CURRENT REVIEW

Ward, B. A. & Gutmann, D. H. Neurofibromatosis 1: from lab bench to clinic. *Pediatr. Neurol.* 2005; **32**:221–228.

SUGGESTED READING

Akenside, M. Observations on cancer. *Med. Trans. Coll. Phys. Lond.* 1785; **1**:64–92.

Barker, D., Wright, E., Nguyen, K. *et al.* Gene for von Recklinghausen NF is in the pericentric region of chromosome 17. *Science* 1987; **236**:1100–1102.

Ferner, R. E. Medical complications of neurofibromatosis. In Huson, S. M., Hughes, R. A. C. (eds). *The Neurofibromatoses. A Pathogenetic and Clinical Overview.* London: Chapman and Hall, 1994; 316–330.

Gutmann, D. A., Aylsworth, A., Carey, J. C. *et al.* The diagnostic evaluation and multi-disciplinary management of neurofibromatosis 1 and neurofibromatosis 2. *J. Am. Med. Assoc.* 1997; **278**:51–58.

Painful double vision and a "hissing" sound

Clinical history

A 50-year-old man described pain behind the left eye during the preceding 10 days as well as a "hissing" tinnitus and double vision. Except for smoking (approximately 30-pack–years), there were no cerebrovascular risk factors or diseases in his medical history.

Examination

On presentation one Thursday afternoon the neurological examination showed left abducens palsy and a pulsatile left orbital bruit. In particular there was no proptosis, ptosis, scleral injection, chemosis or other oculomotor abnormality. The patient reported a recent minor head injury 2 weeks before.

Neurological scores

NIH 0; Barthel Index 100; GCS 15.

Special studies

Cranial CT, visual evoked potentials, visual field test and fundus examination were normal. Ultrasound Doppler duplex showed a higher maximum blood flow velocity of left ICA (1.7 m/s) vs. the right ICA (0.9 m/s), accelerated diastolic flow in both ICAs and abnormal waveforms of flow curves in the left distal ICA and the left carotid siphon. On MRI brain parenchyma was normal. However, MR angiography showed abnormal signal in the region of the cavernous sinuses bilaterally, as well as a striking prominence of the left superior ophthalmic vein.

Follow-up

Over the weekend the patient recovered spontaneously. Ultrasound Doppler duplex showed no extra- or intracranial blood flow acceleration or abnormality any more. Position and velocity of left eye movements in electronystagmography were normal. At this time, the above mentioned findings on MRA had normal-ized. Instead, 3D reconstruction of time-of-flight MR angiography showed a focal aneurysmatic widening of the left ICA which was confirmed a small saccular aneurysm of cavernous part of left ICA on conventional angiography.

Image findings

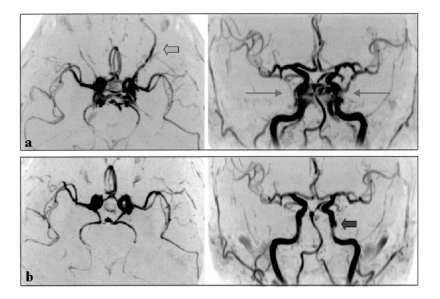

Figure 59.1 3D reconstruction of TOF MRA in axial and coronal plane: (a) initial investigation showed abnormal signal in the region of the cavernous sinuses bilaterally (red arrows), as well as a striking prominence of the left superior ophthalmic vein (green arrow). (b) Three days later, above-mentioned findings had normalized, but bulging of the left ICA was noted (blue arrow). Conventional angiography confirmed a saccular aneurysm of the cavernous part of the left ICA.

Diagnosis

Spontaneous occlusion of carotid cavernous fistula (CCF) with an intracavernous aneurysm of the ICA.

General remarks

CCF can be classified depending on anatomy, etiology and pathophysiology. Based on anatomy, carotid cavernous fistulae are subclassified in direct types (shunt between cavernous portion of ICA and cavernous sinus; type A) and indirect types (shunt between extradural branches of ICA, ECA or both and cavernous sinus; types B–D). Considering aetiology, head trauma (closed or penetrating), (spontaneous or traumatic) rupture of an intracavernous aneurysm of ICA, connective tissue disorders like Ehlers–Danlos syndrome, vascular disease and dural fistulas can be responsible for developing a carotid cavernous fistula. Concerning hemodynamics, carotid cavernous fistulas can show high (mostly type A) or low flow (mostly types B–D).

As a result of the abnormal communications between the arterial and venous system the intravenous pressure rises and the affected veins become arterialized. Stasis of venous and arterial circulation within the eye can cause ocular ischemia and therefore scotoma as well as loss of visual acuity. Increased episcleral pressure may cause increasing intraocular pressure, exophthalmia, scleral injection, and chemosis. By distension and irritation of the third, fourth and sixth cranial nerve embedded in the lateral wall of the cavernous sinus, sudden rise of blood pressure can also lead to diplopia, ptosis, and other oculomotor disturbances. Because of its position close to the ICA vessel wall the sixth cranial nerve (abducens nerve) is affected more often than the other nerves.

Currently, the treatment of choice of a carotid cavernous fistula is an endovascular approach using selective embolisation with detachable platin coils or balloon occlusion. Either an arterial route (through internal carotid artery) or a venous route (through superior ophthalmic vein) can be chosen.

Special remarks

Using the classification mentioned above our patient had a type A, high flow carotid cavernous fistula associated with an aneurysm of the cavernous portion of ICA with spontaneous occlusion, which led to a transient palsy of left abducens nerve. In this special case we were able to completely document the findings with MRA and ultrasound studies before and after occlusion.

SUGGESTED READING

Barrow., D. L, Spector, R. H., Braun, I. F., Landman, J. A., Tindall, S. C., & Tindall, G. T. Classification and treatment of spontaneous carotid cavernous fistulas. *J. Neurosurg.* 1985; **62**:248–256.

Desal, H. A., Toulgoat, F., Racul, S. *et al.* Ehlers–Danlos syndrome type IV and recurrent carotid-cavernous fistula: review of the literature, endovascular approach, technique and difficulties. *Neuroradiology* 2005; **47**:300–304.

Ringer, A. J., Salud, L., & Tomsick, T. A. Carotid cavernous fistulas: anatomy, classification, and treatment. *Neurosurg. Clin. N. Am.* 2005; **16**:279–295.

Spontaneous resolution of PWI/DWI mismatch

Clinical history

A 78-year-old woman presented with fluctuating symptoms over a period of several hours suggestive of left hemispheric ischemia. An hour before coming to the emergency room she developed acute weakness and numbness of the right extremities that lasted several minutes. There were no similar episodes in the past. The history included intermittent atrial fibrillation since 1998, hypertension, and non-insulin-dependent diabetes mellitus. There was no known family history of cardiovascular or cerebrovascular diseases. Current medication included aspirin, propafenol, digoxin, glibenclamide, and monoxidine.

Examination

Clinical examination upon arrival at the hospital was normal. Diagnostic stroke evaluation included an emergency cranial computed tomography, which showed no signs of ischemia, hemorrhage, or of a space-occupying lesion. During this examination the patient suddenly had renewed sensimotor symptoms of the right extremities and a language abnormality consisting of phonematic and semantic paraphasias (NIH 3). The neurologic deficits improved rapidly after the initial MRI within minutes and then remained stable with a discrete aphasia (NIH 1).

Neurological scores

NIH 1; Barthel Index 90; GCS 15.

Special studies

Further evaluation consisted of an emergency MRI, performed 3 hours after initial symptom onset. In the diffusion-weighted images there was an acute lesion in the posterior insular region with corresponding ADC reduction diagnostic for ischemia. There was an extensive perfusion deficit in the left temporo-parietal part of the MCA territory, explained by an M2 occlusion shown in the MR angiography (Fig. 60.1). External and transcranial Doppler examinations performed 5 hours after symptom onset were normal. In particular, there were no signs of vessel stenosis or occlusion of the left middle cerebral artery. The ECG was normal without signs of atrial fibrillation and laboratory values, including those for coagulation disturbances, were likewise within normal limits. Findings of transesophogeal echocardiography were normal and showed no signs of right-to-left shunt. HITS monitoring was negative.

Follow-up

A follow-up MRI performed the next day showed only a small diffusion-weighted lesion in the posterior portion of the insular cortex (Fig. 60.2). There was no remaining perfusion deficit. The patient was placed on warfarin and discharged from the hospital with a discrete aphasia.

Image findings

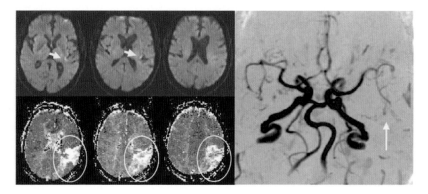

Figure 60.1 MRI performed 3 hours after initial symptom onset: Diffusion-weighted images (*upper left*) show acute ischemic lesion in the posterior insular region, while perfusion MRI (*bottom left*) shows an extensive perfusion deficit in the left middle and posterior MCA territories, corresponding to an M2 occlusion shown in the MR-angiography (right, arrow).

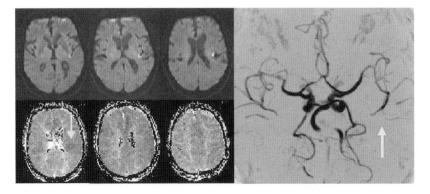

Figure 60.2 MRI performed on the next day shows only the small diffusion-weighted lesion in the insular cortex (*upper left*). Perfusion MRI (*bottom left*) has normalized, a small region shows signs of slight hyperperfusion (arrow) corresponding to recanalization of distal left MCA on MR-angiography.

Diagnosis

Transient MCA occlusion with spontaneous clot resolution.

General remarks

The combination of DWI, PWI and MRA provides a rapid assessment of the ischemic infarct core (DWI), the underlying arterial pathology (MRA) and the tissue at risk (PWI > DWI mismatch). The concept of mismatch, with perfusion larger than diffusion lesion volumes, was postulated as an operational definition of the penumbra by Warach and colleagues in the late 1990s. It has been that the high-intensity signal on DWI identified tissue that usually progresses to complete infarction. The hypoperfused region includes both the severely ischemic core and the at-risk tissue in the mismatch region.

In this case, the initial MRI examination revealed a large perfusion lesion but only minimal DWI abnormality, thereby a large mismatch area. However, the patient did not receive intravenous thrombolysis since the clinical deficit had spontaneously improved after MRI. This was a clinical decision.

Some clinicians, including one of the editors of this volume (LR Caplan), would have given thrombolytics since the future course of the MCA embolus was unknown at the time and thrombolyis would have likely been able to lyse the clot. Thrombolytics lyse clots. In Caplan's mind the key clinical and MRI information include: the location and size of the DWI "infarct," the nature (embolus or in-situ clot), location and severity of the occlusive lesion and the clinical deficit. When the clinical deficit exceeds the DWI lesion (clinical/imaging mismatch), there is brain that is underperfused but not yet infarcted. This brain tissue is at risk of infarction.

Special remarks

This case nicely demonstrates how the PWI–DWI-mismatch concept is a dynamic one. Although rare, spontaneous reopening of vessels may occur and has repeatedly been seen in patients. In such a case the clinical situation needs to be re-evaluated and may – as here – not warrant i.v. thrombolysis.

If this patient had presented with a higher NIH score at the time following the MRI scan, he would have likely received rt-PA on an experimental basis since PWI/DWI mismatch suggests possibly salvageable brain tissue. However, this case shows that spontaneous lysis with both disappearance of perfusion deficits and lack of progression of the diffusion-weighted lesion is possible and likely reflected by clinical signs and symptoms.

SUGGESTED READING

Bardutzky, J., Shen, Q., Bouley, J., Sotak, C. H., Duong, T. Q., & Fisher, M. Perfusion and diffusion imaging in acute focal cerebral ischemia: temporal vs. spatial resolution. *Brain Res.* 2005; **1043**:155–162.

Caplan, L. R. Thrombolysis. *Rev. Neurol. Dis.* 2004; **1**:16–26.

Davalos, A., Blanco, M., Pedraza, S. *et al.* The clinical DWI mismatch: a new diagnostic approach to brain tissue at risk of infarction. *Neurology* 2004; **62**:2187–2192.

Molina, C. A. & Saver, J. L. Extending reperfusion therapy for acute ischemic stroke. *Stroke* 2005; **36**:2311–2320.

Schlaug, G., Benfield, A., Baird, A. E. *et al.* The ischemic penumbra: operationally defined by diffusion and perfusion MRI. *Neurology* 1999; **53**:1528–1537.

Sobesky, J., Zaro Weber, O., Lehnhardt, F. G. *et al.* Does the mismatch match the penumbra? Magnetic resonance imaging and positron emission tomography in early ischemic stroke. *Stroke* 2005; **36**:980–985.

Index